How to Use This Saunders Nursing Survival Guide

This book presents need-to-know information on drug calculations and drug administration in a complete, easy-to-learn format to help you master one of the most difficult subjects in nursing.

These headings walk you through each chapter:

What You WILL LEARN An introductory list of checkpoints to outline what is covered in each chapter.

What It IS A "short and sweet" section devoted to the definition/description of the topic.

What You NEED TO KNOW The essential information and skills to be mastered, with a discussion of why they are important.

What You DO Nursing interventions that apply everything you learned in the What You NEED TO KNOW section.

Do You UNDERSTAND? Various activities and exercises (with answers) so you may review and make sure you understand each topic.

Technical terms (and common hospital terms) are given easy-to-understand explanations, and, if you're likely to hear something referred to in a certain way in the hospital setting, we've highlighted the term in color.

These icons punctuate the text:

 Highlights the most important points to study or use in the clinical atmosphere.

 Alerts you to urgent information about dangerous conditions and how to avoid them.

 Guides you through formulas and problem-solving (with examples).

 Points out age-related variations in signs and symptoms, nursing interventions, and patient teaching.

 Clues you in to possible variations related to a patient's cultural background.

 Instructs you to head to the Internet for additional resources.

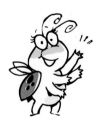

Tell Us What YOU Think

The *Saunders Nursing Survival Guide* series has been created with the help of student feedback to serve your nursing review needs. In order to continue this tradition we invite you to voice your opinion. A website has been created to allow you the opportunity to Tell Us What YOU Think. Please go to the website SNSGSurvey.elsevier.com and help us continue to provide you with student-focused and friendly review activities. Your ideas will be used to create new and fun ways for students like you to learn and review the difficult topics they face throughout their nursing education.

Go to: SNSGSurvey.elsevier.com and Tell Us What YOU Think.

Saunders
Nursing Survival Guide

Drug Calculations
& Drug Administration

Second Edition

Dr. Cynthia Chernecky, PhD, RN, CNS, AOCN
Professor
School of Nursing
Medical College of Georgia
Augusta, Georgia

Mother Helena Infortuna, MTS, BS
Saints Mary and Martha Orthodox Monastery
Wagener, South Carolina

Denise Macklin, BSN, RN, BC
President
Professional Learning Systems, Inc.
Marietta, Georgia

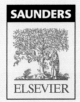

SAUNDERS

ELSEVIER

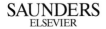

SAUNDERS
ELSEVIER

11830 Westline Industrial Drive
St. Louis, Missouri 63146

SAUNDERS NURSING SURVIVAL GUIDE: ISBN-13: 978-1-4160-2877-2
DRUG CALCULATIONS & DRUG ADMINISTRATION   ISBN-10: 1-4160-2877-3
Copyright © 2006, Elsevier Inc.

Notice

Knowledge and best practice in this field are constantly changing. As new research and experience broaden our knowledge, changes in practice, treatment and drug therapy may become necessary or appropriate. Readers are advised to check the most current information provided (i) on procedures featured or (ii) by the manufacturer of each product to be administered, to verify the recommended dose or formula, the method and duration of administration, and contraindications. It is the responsibility of the practitioner, relying on their own experience and knowledge of the patient, to make diagnoses, to determine dosages and the best treatment for each individual patient, and to take all appropriate safety precautions. To the fullest extent of the law, neither the Publisher nor the Editors assume any liability for any injury and/or damage to persons or property arising out or related to any use of the material contained in this book.

Previous editions copyrighted 2002

ISBN-13: 978-1-4160-2877-2
ISBN-10: 1-4160-2877-3

Acquisitions Editor: Catherine Jackson
Developmental Editor: Amanda Sunderman Politte
Publishing Services Manager: John Rogers
Project Manager: Helen Hudlin
Designer: Jyotika Shroff

Printed in the United States of America

Last digit is the print number: 9   8   7   6   5   4   3   2   1

About the Authors

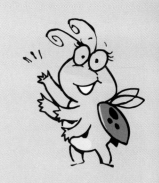

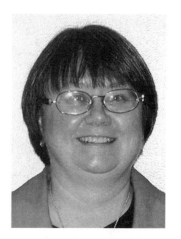

Dr. Cynthia Chernecky earned her degrees at the University of Connecticut (BSN), the University of Pittsburgh (MN), and Case Western Reserve University (PhD). She also earned a NCI fellowship at Yale University and a postdoctorate visiting scholarship at UCLA. Her clinical area of expertise is critical care oncology, with over 23 book publications including *Laboratory Tests and Diagnostic Procedures* (fourth edition) and *Advanced and Critical Care Oncology Nursing: Managing Primary Complications.* She is an international and national speaker, researcher, and published scholar in cancer nursing. She is also active in the Orthodox Church and enjoys life with family, friends, colleagues, and two West Highland white terriers.

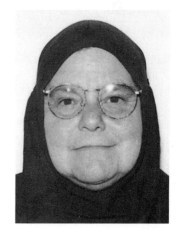

Mother Helena Infortuna was born of immigrant parents in Queens Village, New York. After working in Manhattan as a secretary, she entered the Sisters of Notre Dame de Namur, a teaching order, and was educated at Trinity College in Washington, D.C. While teaching high school mathematics in Pennsylvania, Maryland, New York, and Delaware, she earned her MTS degree from The Catholic University of America and other graduate mathematic credits from Villanova University, the University of Pennsylvania, and the University of Delaware, all through NSF grants. Mother Helena's 37 years in education have included administration as well as teaching. Her first 27 years were in the Catholic school system, followed by 6 years at Newton High School in Elmhurst, a New York city public high school. From there, she moved to Washington, D.C., and taught at both Northern Virginia Community College and Montgomery College. Settling into the Orthodox monastic community of Saints Mary and Martha in Wagener, South Carolina, she taught high school mathematics for 4 more years and currently serves as a private mathematics instructor.

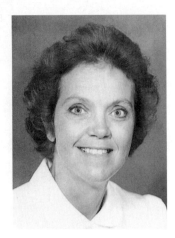

Denise Macklin is President and founder of Professional Learning Systems (PLS), Inc., and the creator and editor-in-chief of *ceuzone.com,* a continuing education Internet site. She is certified in adult/staff education. She has over 25 years of nursing experience (17 years in the specialty of IV therapy). She was included in *Who's Who in Media and Communications 1998* and is a member of the Council of Healthcare Advisors. She is the recipient of the Suzanne Hurbst award for vascular access, a research grant related to vascular access education from the National Institute for Nursing Research. Denise has lectured around the United States on a wide variety of topics related to IV therapy and has published articles in various publications, including the *American Journal of Nursing, Journal of Intravenous Nursing, Journal of Vascular Access Devices,* and *Nursing Management and Dimensions of Critical Care.* She is a contributing author to Saunders *Manual of Medical-Surgical Nursing: A Guide to Clinical Decision Making* and co-author of *Fluids & Electrolytes* and *IV Therapy* in this book series and *Math for Clinical Practice.* Her work includes extensive experience in the production of training videos for vascular access and interactive programs for medical manufacturers and the CDC. PLS's videos, CD-I programs, and web CE offerings are being used to educate nurses not only in the United States but also in Canada, England, mainland Europe, Turkey, and several countries on the Pacific rim.

Contributors to the First Edition

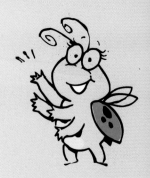

Jeanette Adams, PhD, RN, MS, CRNI, CS
Consultant
Mercer Island, Washington

Jane Brazy, MD
Neonatologist and Professor of Pediatrics
University of Wisconsin Medical School
Madison, Wisconsin

Diane Cope, PhD, RN, AOCN
Nurse Practitioner
Private Practice in Oncology
Fort Meyers, Florida

Christine Marie Fong, MD
Neonatologist
Meriter Hospital
Madison, Wisconsin

Michelle Frey, RN, MS, AOCN
Administrative Director of Children's Services
Consulting Associate at the Duke University School
    of Nursing
Duke University Medical Center
Durham, North Carolina

Mary Ann Ihlenfeld, RN, BSN
Staff Nurse, Oncology
Meriter Hospital
Madison, Wisconsin

Barbara S. Kiernan, PhD, RN, CS, PNP
Assistant Professor of Nursing, Parent-Child
    Nursing
Medical College of Georgia
School of Nursing
Augusta, Georgia

Collette L. McKinney, MSN, RN
OIC, Urgent Care Center
Bassett Army Community Hospital
Fort Wainwright, Alaska

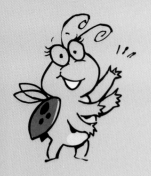

Faculty & Student Reviewers for the First Edition

FACULTY

Luvencia Connor, RN
Pediatric Nurse
Memorial Hospital West
Pembroke Pines, Florida

Eileen Marie Griffiths, MSN, RN
Miami-Dade Community College
Miami, Florida

Shirley A. Hemminger, MSN, RN, CCRN
Instructor
Kent State College of Nursing
Kent, Ohio
Staff Nurse
University Hospitals of Cleveland
Cleveland, Ohio

Joyce LeFever Kee, MS, RN
Associate Professor Emerita
College of Health and Nursing Sciences
University of Delaware
Newark, Delaware

Dorothy B. Liddel, MSN, RN, ONC
Retired Associate Professor of Nursing
Bethesda, Maryland

Mary Ellen Mitchell-Rosen, BSN
Instructor
Deck Department
RTM Simulation Training and Research Center
Dania Beach, Florida

Michelle A. Mongillo, RN, BSN, CRRN
Independent Nurse Consultant
Coral Springs, Florida

Michael Tomak, RN, BSN
Assistant Professor
Miami-Dade Community College
Miami, Florida

STUDENTS

Kimberly Ann Bloom
Bloomsburg University
Bloomsburg, Pennsylvania

Lori Burton
Medical College of Georgia
School of Nursing
Athens, Georgia

Lorrie Kirby, CNA
Austin Community College
Austin, Texas

Melissa Schondelmayer
Medical College of Georgia
School of Nursing
Athens, Georgia

Series Reviewers

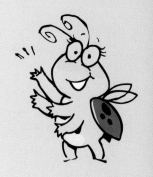

FACULTY

Edwina A. McConnell, PhD, RN, FRCNA
Professor
School of Nursing
Texas Technical University Health Sciences Center
Lubbock, Texas
Consultant
Gorham, Maine

Judith L. Myers, MSN, RN
Health Sciences Center
St. Louis University School of Nursing
St. Louis, Missouri

STUDENTS

Joy Kutlenios Amos, RN, BSN
Piedmont Medical Center
Rock Hill, South Carolina
Former student
Wheeling Jesuit University
Wheeling, West Virginia

Angela M. Boyd, AS
University of Tennessee at Martin
Martin, Tennessee

Shayne Michael Gray, RN, BSN
University of Arkansas
Little Rock, Arkansas

Jill Hall, RN
Miller Children's Hospital
Long Beach, California

Jennifer Hamilton
University of Virginia
Charlottesville, Virginia

Elizabeth J. Hoogmoed, RN, BSN
Valley Hospital
Ridgewood, New Jersey

Katie Scarlett McRae, BA, BSN
Oregon Health Sciences University
Portland, Oregon

Preface

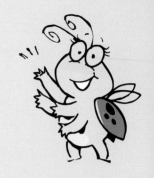

The goal of nursing is to assist in the attainment of positive outcomes when caring for people with health problems. This requires a depth of knowledge for safe and effective care, including one particularly important responsibility—the administration of medications. This book will help you master the challenges of correctly calculating prescribed dosages and safely administering drugs in an effort to avoid human error.

The *Saunders Nursing Survival Guide* series was created with your input. Nursing students told us about the topics they found more difficult to master, such as dosage calculations, fluids and electrolytes, ECGs, IV therapy, critical care and emergency nursing, and hemodynamic monitoring. Focus groups were held at the National Student Nurses Association meeting, and we asked you what would be the best way to learn this difficult material. Your responses were certainly interesting! You said we should keep the text to a minimum; use an engaging, fun approach; provide ample space to write on the pages; include a variety of activities to appeal to students with different learning styles; make the content visually appealing; and provide NCLEX review questions so you could check your understanding of key topics and perform any necessary review. The *Saunders Nursing Survival Guide* series is the result of your ideas.

The chapters in *Drug Calculations & Drug Administration* progress from a general review of basic mathematical principles (Part I) to more advanced topics that will help you deal with changing technologies and special populations (Part IV). The "meat" of the book (Parts II and III) instructs you on all methods of drug administration. Because of the many complexities of intravenous administration, we chose to cover it in its own section (Part III).

We include many features in the margins to help you focus on the vital information you'll need to succeed in the classroom and in the clinical setting. The TAKE HOME POINTS icon offers both study tips for classroom tests and "pearls of wisdom" to assist you in caring for patients. Both are drawn from our many years of combined academic and clinical experience. The CAUTION icon is vital and usually involves nursing actions that may have life-threatening consequences. The LIFE SPAN icon and the CULTURE icon highlight variations in treatment that may be necessary for specific age or ethnic groups. A CALCULATOR icon will draw your eye to important equations and examples that will help you calculate proper medication dosages. A WEB LINKS icon will direct you to sites on the Internet that give more detailed information on a given topic.

We also use consistent headings that emphasize specific nursing actions. *What You WILL LEARN* provides a list of the concepts to be learned in that chapter. *What It IS* provides a definition of the topic. *What You NEED TO KNOW* gives you all the current information necessary to plan quality care, and *What You DO* explains what you do as a practicing nurse. Finally, *Do You UNDERSTAND* provides questions and exercises that are both entertaining and useful to reinforce the topic's concepts. We hope you will find reading this book and completing the activities as fun as creating the content was!

It is because of the knowledge and understanding of drug dosages and administration that, despite daily stressors, nurses continue to provide effective care for persons in a respectful and competent manner. It is our professional responsibility to learn and to continue our journey toward this goal. It's a hard road to travel—may this book guide you on your way.

Acknowledgements

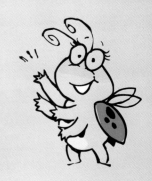

I would like to thank from my heart the co-editors of this book, who tackled the project with fervor, faith, and fondness of heart. (Naturally, a few walks to clear my mind and a glass of wine to soothe my soul didn't hurt either!) It is with trust and teamwork that we were able to create a book that will help future and current nurses learn to care in a truthful and effective manner. Thanks to each of you for your professional commitment. I would also like to thank those who supported us in this project: the professional personnel at Elsevier; my mother Olga and Godmother Helen Prohorik; colleagues Dr. Ann Marie Kolanowski, Dr. Marlene Rosenkoetter, Dr. Linda Sarna, Dr. Leda Danao, Molly Loney, Pam Cushman, Nancy Stark, Rebecca Rule, Dr. Jean Brown, Dr. Mary Cooley, Dr. Geri Padilla; and Mother Thecla, Mother Helena, and Mother Seraphina of Saints Mary and Martha Orthodox Monastery.

—*Dr. Cynthia (Cinda) Chernecky*

I would like to give praise and thanks to our good God for His many gifts and for bringing such wonderful people into my life, among them Dr. Cynthia Chernecky, without whom this book would not exist.

—*Mother Helena Infortuna*

I would like to thank my co-editors of this book. Their dedication to education and the generosity of their spirit has been invaluable to me. I would like to thank the many people at Elsevier who supported this book. Without their efforts this book would never have been produced. I would like to thank my husband, Dana, who has supported me though-out this book as well as my many other professional endeavors. Without strong family support, professional success is not attainable.

—*Denise Macklin*

Mathematics Review

What You WILL LEARN

After reading this chapter, you will know how to do the following:

- ✔ Recognize the necessity of the use of relative value in application to clinical care.
- ✔ Perform computations of addition, subtraction, multiplication, and division.
- ✔ Express and convert fractions, ratios, and percentages.
- ✔ Appropriately determine proportions and ratios for solving clinical problems.
- ✔ Calculate percentages as they apply to clinical needs.

The *decimal point* is the first mathematics topic reviewed. There are five concepts to understand: (1) relative value, (2) addition, (3) subtraction, (4) multiplication, and (5) division.

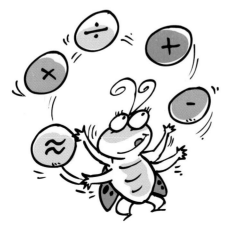

What IS the Relative Value of a Decimal?

You will need to recognize the high and low values of a decimal number and understand its value to calculate doses. The following illustrates a series of digits with a value:

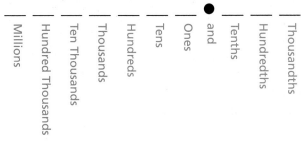

Write the following decimal number in the space provided: one million, two hundred thirty-four thousand, five hundred sixty-seven, and eighty-nine hundredths.

_____ . _____

Answer: 1,234,567.89

What You NEED TO KNOW

The *relative value* of the number is determined by the spaces left of the decimal point—the more spaces, the higher the value. When comparing numbers with the same quantity of spaces to the left of a decimal point, the first place where they differ determines the relative value of each number.

What You DO

EXAMPLE 1: **Which is the higher value? 24.35**
(twenty-four and thirty-five hundredths)
or 25.2 (twenty-five and two tenths)

To compare numbers:

• Write the numbers with each decimal point aligned.

  a. 24.35

  b. 25.2

• Beginning with the first number (where the highest value begins) and
moving to the right, identify the first place where the numbers differ.

• They differ at the second place from the left (numbers 4 and 5).

• The larger number determines the higher value.

• 25.2 is the higher of the two numbers and therefore the answer.

EXAMPLE 2: **Which is the higher value? 0.34 or 0.335**

  a. 0.34

  b. 0.335

Answer: 0.34

EXAMPLE 3: **Identify the highest value.**

  a. 4.55

  b. 4.5

  c. 4.375

Determine the value that can be eliminated. Options *a* and *b* are obvi-
ously higher values than option *c*. Drop option *c* from consideration, and
compare the remaining two numbers.

  a. 4.55

  b. 4.5

Answer: 4.55

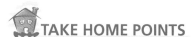

TAKE HOME POINTS

To determine relative value:
1. Line up each of the numbers
   with one decimal point under
   the other decimal point.
2. Look for the first place from
   the left where the numbers
   differ.

EXAMPLE 4: **The prescription reads to administer an oral dose of 0.125 mg digoxin now. The digoxin tablets on hand have a strength of 0.25 mg. How many tablets of digoxin should you give now?**

a. 1 tablet
b. Less than 1 tablet
c. More than 1 tablet

Answer: Less than 1 tablet

Fill in the proper dose for Example 4.

Do You UNDERSTAND?

DIRECTIONS: **Circle the number with the highest value in each problem.**

1. (a) 3.5;   (b) 2.75;   (c) 3.55
2. (a) 1.5;   (b) 1.35;   (c) 1.25
3. (a) 0.95;   (b) 0.925;   (c) 0.975

What IS Addition?

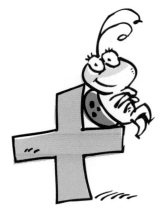

The mathematical operation of combining numbers to determine their accumulative value is *addition*. The result is called the *sum*.

What You NEED TO KNOW

To find the sum of decimal numbers, write each number so that their decimal points are aligned. Add the numbers beginning from the right column and continuing to the left, placing the decimal point in the answer under the other decimal points.

What You DO

EXAMPLE 1: **1.23 + 22.45 = 23.68**

To add decimal numbers:
- Write each number, aligning the decimal points.

    1.23
  22.45

- Beginning at the right, add each column (add 3 and 5, 2 and 4, 1 and 2, and 0 and 2).

$$
\begin{array}{cccccc}
0 & 1 & . & 2 & 3 \\
2 & 2 & . & 4 & 5 \\
\hline
2 & 3 & . & 6 & 8
\end{array}
$$

- Remember to include the decimal point in your answer.

EXAMPLE 2: **0.55 + 0.375**

    1
   0.55
+ 0.375
──────
  0.925

- Remember, if the sum of the numbers in a column is 10 or greater, add the tens digit to the next column to the left.

EXAMPLE 3: **1.05 + 2.3 + 0.75**

  1 1
 1.05
 2.3
+ 0.75
──────
 4.10

EXAMPLE 4: **A patient receives four medications: 0.2 mg, 1.5 mg, 0.75 mg, and 2 mg. What is the total dose?**

  1
 0.2
 1.5
 0.75
+ 2.
──────
 4.45 mg

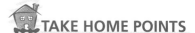

TAKE HOME POINTS

To add decimal numbers:
1. Write the numbers, aligning the decimal points.
2. Begin adding with the right column.
3. Align the decimal point in your answer with the above points.

Do You UNDERSTAND?

DIRECTIONS: Add the following numbers:
1. 1.25 + 1.5 = _____
2. 0.35 + 1.275 = _____
3. 11.3 + 1.45 = _____
4. 12.5 mg Demerol + 0.4 mg atropine = _____
5. Audrey receives daily medication doses of 0.5 mg at breakfast, 0.5 mg and 0.25 mg at lunch, and 0.75 mg at dinner. How many milligrams does Audrey consume each day?

What IS Subtraction?

Subtraction is the opposite mathematical operation of addition. Instead of combining numbers to increase their total value, the numbers are combined to decrease their total value. The result is called the *difference*.

What You NEED TO KNOW

To determine the difference between decimal numbers, write each number with the decimal points aligned. If there are different numbers of digits to the right of the decimal point, it may be helpful to add zeros to the shorter numbers to make all numbers equally long. Begin subtraction from the right column and continue to the left, placing the decimal point in the answer under the other decimal points.

Answers: 1. 2.75; 2. 1.625; 3. 12.75; 4. 12.9 mg; 5. 2.0 mg.

What You DO

EXAMPLE 1: 2.55 – 0.2

To subtract decimal numbers:
- Write the numbers, aligning the decimal points.

  2.55
  0.2
- Add zeros as necessary.

  2.55
  0.20
- Beginning with the right column, subtract the bottom number from the top (subtract 0 from 5, 2 from 5, and 0 from 2).

$$
\begin{array}{r}
2\ .\ 5\ \ 5 \\
-\,0\ .\ 2\ \ 0 \\
\hline
2\ .\ 3\ \ 5
\end{array}
$$
- Align the decimal point in your answer with the above points.

The following examples illustrate how to solve a problem when the digit being subtracted is greater than the digit above it.

EXAMPLE 2: 1.54 – 0.325

  1.540
  0.325

Since 5 is greater than 0, change the 4 hundredths to 3 hundredths and increase the 0 thousandth to 10 thousandths. Subtract 5 from 10, 2 from 3, 3 from 5, and 0 from 1.

$$
\begin{array}{r}
^{3\,10} \\
1.5\cancel{4}\cancel{0} \\
-\,0.325 \\
\hline
1.215
\end{array}
$$

EXAMPLE 3: 3.2 – 0.65

$$
\begin{array}{r}
^{2}\quad ^{11}\quad ^{10} \\
\cancel{3}\ .\ \cancel{2}\ \ \cancel{0} \\
-\,0\ .\ 6\ \ 5 \\
\hline
2\ .\ 5\ \ 5
\end{array}
$$

EXAMPLE 4: **The patient needs a dose of 9.5 mg. You have one tablet of 4.75 mg. How many more milligrams must you give?**

$$
\begin{array}{ccc}
8 & 14 & 10 \\
\cancel{9} & .\ \cancel{5} & \cancel{0} \\
-4 & .\ 7 & 5 \\
\hline
4 & .\ 7 & 5 \text{ mg}
\end{array}
$$

TAKE HOME POINTS

To subtract decimal numbers:
1. Write the numbers, aligning the decimal points.
2. Add zeros to make the same number of digits to the right of the decimal point.
3. If the top digit is lesser in value than the bottom digit, reduce the top digit immediately to the left by 1 and add 10 to the right top digit.
4. Beginning with the right column, subtract the bottom number from the top number.
5. Align the decimal point in your answer with the above points.

Do You UNDERSTAND?

DIRECTIONS: **Subtract the following numbers to find the differences:**
1. 0.3 − 0.07 = _____
2. 12.5 − 1.25 = _____
3. 4.25 − 2.35 = _____
4. How many tablets will you need to prepare a dose of 4.8 mg using 1.6 mg tablets? _____
5. A prescribed dosage reads 1000 mg (1 g) Cipro (ciprofloxacin) in a 24-hour period. Mr. Chang has received 250 mg. How many more milligrams must he take to complete the prescribed dosage?

_____

What IS Multiplication?

The mathematical operation of repeated addition is referred to as *multiplication*. The result is called the *product*.

What You NEED TO KNOW

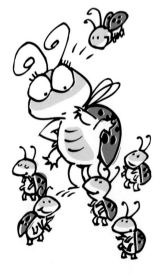

To find the *product* of decimal numbers, the placement of the decimal point in the answer is crucial. The number of decimal places in the product is the sum of the decimal places in each of the numbers being multiplied.

Answers: 1. 0.23; 2. 11.25; 3. 1.90; 4. 3 tablets; 5. 750 mg.

What You DO

EXAMPLE 1: 2.3 × 0.25

To multiply decimal numbers:
- Multiply as with any whole numbers.

      2.3
    × 0.25

- First multiply 23 by 5 and then 23 by 2.

        1
      2.3
    × 0.25
    ─────
      115   (product of 23 × 5)
    + 46   (product of 23 × 2)
    ─────
      575   (sum of each product)

- Decide how many decimal places are needed in your answer by adding the number of decimal places to the right of the decimal point in each number.

    2.3
    0.25 (three places to the right of the decimal points)

- Count the number of places from right to left (5, 7, 5); place the decimal point in your answer.

    Answer: 0 . 5 7 5

EXAMPLE 2: 0.32 × 0.17

      0.32
    × 0.17
    ─────
      224
    + 32
    ─────
    0544

There are two decimal places to the right of the decimal point in both 0.32 and 0.17. Four decimal places are needed in the product.

    Answer: 0 . 0 5 4 4

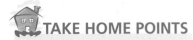
TAKE HOME POINTS

Placement of the decimal point is crucial in multiplication.
To multiply decimal numbers:
1. Multiply the numbers as if they were whole numbers.
2. Add the number of places to the right of the decimal points in both numbers, and place a decimal point the same number of places to the left in your answer.

EXAMPLE 3: 6.25×1.5

$$
\begin{array}{r}
6.25 \\
\times 1.5 \\
\hline
3125 \\
+ 625 \\
\hline
9375
\end{array}
$$

Answer: 9 . 3 7 5

EXAMPLE 4: You are asked to administer four tablets with the strength of 0.04 mg each. What is the total dose?

$$
\begin{array}{r}
0.04 \\
\times \quad 4 \\
\hline
016
\end{array}
$$

Answer: 0 . 1 6 mg

Do You UNDERSTAND?

DIRECTIONS: **Multiply the following:**
1. $4 \times 3.15 =$ _____
2. $1.5 \times 0.05 =$ _____
3. $1.25 \times 0.35 =$ _____
4. The tablets available for your patient are labeled 12.5 mg, and you have been asked to administer 3½ (3.5) tablets. What is the total dose given?

What IS Division?

Division is the opposite mathematical operation of multiplication. Instead of repeated addition, division is repeated subtraction.

Answers: 1. 12.6; 2. 0.075; 3. 0.4375; 4. 43.75 mg.

Division is written using several symbols, such as 1 ÷ 2, 2)$\overline{1}$, or ½. The *divisor* (the number performing the division) is on the right of the first symbol, the left of the second symbol, and the bottom of the third symbol. The answer to a division problem is called the *quotient*.

What You NEED TO KNOW

To find the *quotient* of decimal numbers, the divisor must be a whole number (a number with no decimal point) and the decimal point must be correctly placed in the answer. When a decimal number is being divided by a whole number, the decimal point is placed directly above the decimal point in the *dividend* (number being divided). When a number is being divided by a decimal number, the decimal point in the divisor must be moved to the right as many places as necessary to make the divisor a whole number. The decimal point in the dividend must be moved the same number of places to the right. The decimal point in the quotient is placed directly above the new position of the decimal point in the dividend.

What You DO

EXAMPLE 1: 3.25 ÷ 0.5

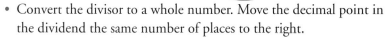

To divide decimal numbers:

- Convert the divisor to a whole number. Move the decimal point in the dividend the same number of places to the right.

  0 . 5)$\overline{3 . 2\ 5}$

- Place the decimal point in the quotient directly above its new position in the dividend.

  5)$\overline{32.5}$

- Perform the calculation.

$$
\begin{array}{r}
6.5 \\
5\overline{)32.5} \\
30 \\
\hline
2\,5 \\
2\,5 \\
\hline
0
\end{array}
$$

EXAMPLE 2: 4.10 ÷ 2.05.
Convert the divisor to a whole number (205), and move the decimal in the dividend (4.10) the same number of spaces (410). Place the decimal point accurately in the quotient.

$$
\begin{array}{r}
2.0 \\
205\overline{)410.0} \\
410 \\
\hline
0
\end{array}
$$

EXAMPLE 3: 0.25 ÷ 0.15 (25 ÷ 15)

$$
\begin{array}{r}
1.66 \\
015\overline{)025.00} \\
15 \\
\hline
100 \\
90 \\
\hline
100 \\
90 \\
\hline
10
\end{array}
$$

Since there will be a remainder, round the quotient to 1.7. To round a number to an indicated decimal place, look at the digit to the right of it. If it is 5 or greater, increase the digit by 1. If the digit is less than 5, leave the indicated digit as is.

EXAMPLE 4: Your patient is to receive a dose of 3.75 mg. The tablets available are labeled 1.5 mg. How many tablets should you place in the medicine drawer?

$$
\begin{array}{r}
2.5 (2\tfrac{1}{2}) \text{ tablets} \\
15\overline{)37.5} \\
30 \\
\hline
75 \\
75 \\
\hline
0
\end{array}
$$

TAKE HOME POINTS

To divide decimal numbers:
1. Convert the divisor to a whole number (if necessary) by shifting the decimal point to the right.
2. Move the decimal point in the dividend the same number of places to the right.
3. Place the decimal point in the quotient directly above its new position in the dividend.
4. Round the answer, if necessary.

Do You UNDERSTAND?

DIRECTIONS: **Divide the following:**
1. $3.75 \div 3 =$ _____
2. $5 \div 2.25 =$ _____
3. $12.35 \div 3.25 =$ _____
4. Your patient is to receive a total dose of 3.75 mg of medication. Available tablets are labeled 2.5 mg. How many tablets are needed?

Having completed a review of the concepts of decimals that are necessary to calculate medication doses, the following text provides a review of fractions. These concepts include multiplying and dividing fractions, solving equations, and working with ratios and proportions.

What IS a Fraction?

A *fraction* is a mathematical expression comparing two numbers by division. The top number is called the *numerator,* and the bottom number is called the *denominator.*

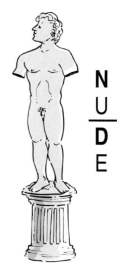

$$\frac{N\ U}{D\ E}$$

A good way to remember that the *numerator* is the top number and the *denominator* is the bottom number is that "Nu" on top and "De" on the bottom spell "Nude."

What You NEED TO KNOW

The relative value of two or more fractions is determined in one of the following ways:
• If the denominators are the same, the fraction with the *highest numerator* has the *highest value.*
• If the numerators are the same, the fraction with the *lowest denominator* has the *highest value.*
• If each fraction is written as its decimal equivalent (by performing the indicated division), the fraction with the *highest decimal number* has the *highest value.*

What You DO

EXAMPLE 1: In each of the following problems, identify the fraction with the highest value:

1. ³/₈, ¹/₈, ⁵/₈
   - Since the denominators are the same, ⁵/₈ has the highest value because 5 is the highest numerator.
2. ³/₄, ³/₅, ³/₆
   - Since the numerators are the same, ³/₄ has the highest value because 4 is the lowest denominator.
3. ¹/₂, ³/₄, ²/₃
   - Since ¹/₂ = 1 ÷ 2 or $2\overline{)1.0}$ = 0.5, ³/₄ = 3 ÷ 4 = 0.75, and ²/₃ = 2 ÷ 3 = 0.67, ³/₄ is the highest value because 0.75 is the highest decimal value.

TAKE HOME POINTS

To determine the relative value of fractions:
1. If the denominators are the same, the highest numerator determines the highest fraction.
2. If the numerators are the same, the lowest denominator determines the highest fraction.
   OR
3. Convert each fraction to its decimal equivalent by dividing the numerator (top number) by the denominator (bottom number) and comparing the decimal numbers.

Do You UNDERSTAND?

DIRECTIONS: In each of the following problems, identify the fraction that has the highest value:

1. (a) ¹/₁₂;   (b) ¹/₈;   (c) ¹/₁₀
2. (a) ²/₈;   (b) ¹/₈;   (c) ⁴/₈
3. (a) ²/₅;   (b) ¹/₈;   (c) ⁵/₆
4. You have tablets that are ¹/₆ strength of the whole, but your patient needs ¹/₂ strength. What should be administered to your patient?
   a. Less than 1 tablet
   b. More than 1 tablet
5. Manny is in charge of getting a snack for a party during his shift. There are several party platters on sale at his local grocery store for exactly the same price. The first platter has a ²/₃-wedge of sharp cheddar cheese; a second platter has a ⁶/₇-wedge of Swiss cheese, and a third platter has a ³/₄-wedge of colby cheese. If all these cheese blocks were equal in size when whole, which platter should Manny buy to have the most cheese for the people at the party?

What IS Multiplication of Fractions?

As previously mentioned, the mathematical operation of repeated addition is referred to as *multiplication*. The result is called the *product*.

What You NEED TO KNOW

To calculate doses, reduce the numbers (i.e., divide both the numerator and the denominator by the same number), when possible. Multiply the remaining numerators and the remaining denominators. The resulting fraction is the answer. (It is sometimes necessary to change the solution to its decimal equivalent by dividing the numerator by the denominator.)

What You DO

EXAMPLE 1: $\frac{1}{6} \times \frac{3}{4} = \frac{1}{8}$
To multiply fraction numbers:
- Reduce the fractions when possible as shown. Determine whether the fractions have numerators and denominators that can be divided by the same number.

$$\frac{1}{\overset{}{\underset{2}{6}}} \times \frac{\overset{1}{\cancel{3}}}{4}$$

The denominator of the first fraction and numerator of the second fraction are both divisible by 3.
- Multiply the remaining numerators; multiply the remaining denominators.

$$\frac{1}{2} \times \frac{1}{4} = \frac{1}{8}$$

- Express the final answer as a decimal to the nearest tenth.

0.125 or 0.1 (See previous discussion on rounding.)

$$\frac{1}{8} = 8\overline{)1.000}$$

$$\begin{array}{r} \underline{8} \\ 20 \\ \underline{16} \\ 40 \\ \underline{40} \\ 0 \end{array}$$

EXAMPLE 2: $\frac{1}{6} \times \frac{4}{3}$

$$\frac{1}{\overset{}{\underset{3}{\cancel{6}}}} \times \frac{\overset{2}{\cancel{4}}}{3}$$

The denominator of the first fraction and numerator of the second fraction are both divisible by 2.

$$\frac{1}{3} \times \frac{2}{3} = \frac{2}{9}$$

0.22 = 0.2 (rounded to the nearest tenth)

$$9\overline{)2.00}$$

$$\begin{array}{r} \underline{18} \\ 20 \\ \underline{18} \\ 2 \end{array}$$

TAKE HOME POINTS

To multiply fractions:
1. Reduce when possible.
2. Multiply the remaining numerators; multiply the remaining denominators.
3. Change the product to a decimal when necessary.

EXAMPLE 3: $\frac{1}{3} \times \frac{4}{1} = \frac{4}{3}$ **(The numerator and denominator are not both divisible by a number.)**

1.33 = 1.3 (rounded to the nearest tenth)

$$3\overline{)4.00}$$

$$\begin{array}{r} \underline{3} \\ 10 \\ \underline{9} \\ 10 \\ \underline{9} \\ 1 \end{array}$$

Do You UNDERSTAND?

DIRECTIONS: **Multiply the following:**

1. $\frac{1}{8} \times \frac{6}{1} =$ _____
2. $\frac{1}{2} \times \frac{1}{3} =$ _____
3. $\frac{1}{50} \times \frac{100}{1} =$ _____
4. $\frac{7}{8} \times \frac{2}{21} =$ _____

What IS Division of Fractions?

The *division* of fractions is accomplished by multiplying by the *reciprocal* of the *divisor*.

What You NEED TO KNOW

To find the *reciprocal* of a fraction, transpose the numerator (top) and denominator (bottom) of the fraction. (This is also called *inverting the fraction*.) To divide fractions, keep the first fraction as is and multiply by the reciprocal of the divisor. In dose calculations, division of two fractions is usually indicated by a fraction line rather than the division symbol (÷).

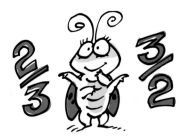

FRACTION   RECIPROCAL

What You DO

EXAMPLE 1: $\dfrac{3/4}{1/2}$

To divide these two fractions:

- Leave the numerator fraction as $3/4$.
- Determine the reciprocal of the denominator fraction ($1/2$).

- Multiply the two fractions. (See previous section on multiplying fractions.)

$$\frac{3}{\overset{}{\underset{2}{4}}} \times \frac{\overset{1}{\cancel{2}}}{1} = \frac{3}{2}$$

$$\begin{array}{r} 1.5 \\ 2\overline{)3.0} \\ \underline{2} \\ 10 \\ \underline{10} \\ 0 \end{array}$$

EXAMPLE 2: $\dfrac{1/8}{1/4}$

$$\frac{1}{\underset{2}{\cancel{8}}} \times \frac{\overset{1}{\cancel{4}}}{1} = \frac{1}{2}$$

$$\begin{array}{r} .5 \\ 2\overline{)1.0} \\ \underline{10} \\ 0 \end{array}$$

EXAMPLE 3: $\dfrac{1/75}{1/150}$

$$\frac{1}{\underset{1}{\cancel{75}}} \times \frac{\overset{2}{\cancel{150}}}{1} = \frac{2}{1}$$

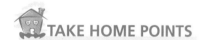TAKE HOME POINTS

To divide fractions:
1. Keep the first fraction as written.
2. Determine the reciprocal of the divisor (transpose the numerator and denominator).
3. Multiply the fractions, reducing when possible.
4. Convert the result to a decimal if useful.

EXAMPLE 4: You have been asked to administer morphine sulfate gr ¹⁄6. The supply of morphine sulfate tablets is labeled gr ¹⁄4. How many tablets will you use?

$$\frac{1}{6} \div \frac{1}{4} = \frac{1}{\underset{3}{\cancel{6}}} \times \frac{\overset{2}{\cancel{4}}}{1} = \frac{2}{3} \text{ tablet}$$

Do You UNDERSTAND?

DIRECTIONS: **Divide the following fractions:**

1. $\dfrac{^1/_{250}}{^1/_{100}}$ = _____

2. $\dfrac{^1/_{10}}{^1/_6}$ = _____

3. $\dfrac{^2/_3}{^1/_4}$ = _____

4. You are asked to administer gr $^1/_3$ codeine phosphate. Available tablets are labeled gr $^1/_6$ codeine phosphate. How many tablets should be given?

_____

What IS Solving an Equation?

An *equation* is a mathematical sentence that contains an equal sign (=) and a letter or an unknown entity known as a *variable*. The solution to an equation is a value that makes the sentence true.

What You NEED TO KNOW

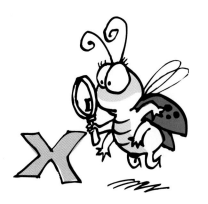

In calculating doses, you will be required to determine the value of an unknown (x).

What You DO

EXAMPLE 1: Determine the value of x if $x = 300 \times {}^1/_{60}$

To determine the value of the x variable (reduce fractions; multiply remaining numerators and denominators):

$$x = \frac{\overset{5}{\cancel{300}}}{1} \times \frac{1}{\underset{1}{\cancel{60}}} = 5$$

Answer: $x = 5$

EXAMPLE 2: $x = {}^{75}/_{50} \times 4$

$$x = \frac{\overset{3}{\cancel{75}}}{\underset{\underset{1}{\cancel{25}}}{\cancel{50}}} \times \frac{\overset{2}{\cancel{4}}}{1} = \frac{3}{1} \times \frac{2}{1} = 6$$

Answer: $x = 6$

EXAMPLE 3: $x = {}^{375}/_{250} \times 3$

$$x = \frac{\overset{15}{\cancel{375}}}{\underset{10}{\cancel{250}}} \times \frac{3}{1} = \frac{45}{10} = 4.5$$

Answer: $x = 4.5$

EXAMPLE 4: $x = {}^{0.5}/_{1.35} \times 1.5$

Eliminate decimal points from a fraction by moving the decimal point an equal number of places to the right in both the numerator and the denominator.

$$\frac{0.5}{1.35} = \frac{50}{135} \quad \text{and} \quad \frac{1.5}{1} = \frac{15}{10}$$

$$x = \frac{\overset{5}{\cancel{50}}}{\underset{9}{\cancel{135}}} \times \frac{\overset{1}{\cancel{15}}}{\underset{1}{\cancel{10}}} = \frac{5}{9} = 0.55$$

Answer: $x = 0.6$ (rounded to the nearest tenth)

EXAMPLE 5: $x = \dfrac{^{1}/_{120}}{^{2}/_{150}} \times 3$

$$x = \dfrac{1}{\underset{4}{\cancel{120}}} \times \dfrac{\overset{5}{\cancel{150}}}{2} \times \dfrac{3}{1}$$

$$x = \dfrac{1}{4} \times \dfrac{5}{2} \times \dfrac{3}{1} = \dfrac{15}{8} = 1.87$$

Answer: $x = 1.9$ (rounded to the nearest tenth)

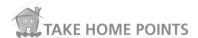

TAKE HOME POINTS

To determine the value of the x variable:
1. Reduce the numbers when possible.
2. Multiply the remaining numerators.
3. Multiply the remaining denominators.
4. Divide the numerator by the denominator.
5. Round the answer to the nearest tenth.

Do You UNDERSTAND?

DIRECTIONS: **Determine the value of x.**

1. $x = {}^{250}/_{1000} \times 1.2 = $ _____

2. $x = {}^{20}/_{30} \times 2 = $ _____

3. $x = {}^{1,200,000}/_{900,000} \times 3.5 = $ _____

4. $x = {}^{0.25}/_{1.5} \times 1.3 = $ _____

5. $x = \dfrac{^{1}/_{100}}{^{1}/_{150}} \times 2.3 = $ _____

What IS a Ratio?

A *ratio* is a comparison of two quantities using division. Division may be indicated by either a colon or a fraction line (e.g., 1:100 or $^{1}/_{100}$).

What You NEED TO KNOW

Ratios are commonly used to express the relationship between the weight (strength) of a drug and a tablet or capsule. In the case of liquid medication, ratios express the relationship between the weight of a drug and the volume of the solution.

What You Do

EXAMPLE 1: **A capsule contains 250 mg, which is written as either 1 capsule/250 mg or 250 mg/capsule.**

EXAMPLE 2: **A solution that contains 250 mg in each 1.5 mL solution may be written as 250 mg/1.5 mL or 1.5 mL/250 mg.**

EXAMPLE 3: **A 2 mL solution that contains 150 mg may be written as 2 mL/150 mg or 150 mg/2 mL.**

EXAMPLE 4: **A tablet that contains 50 mg may be written as 50 mg/1 tablet or 1 tablet/50 mg.**

TAKE HOME POINTS

To express doses as ratios, include the units of measure with the numeric values.

Do You UNDERSTAND?

DIRECTIONS: Express the following doses as ratios:
1. A tablet contains 0.4 mg medication.
2. An injection contains 100 mg in each mL solution.
3. A capsule contains 450 mg medication.
4. An injection contains 500 mg in each 0.7 mL solution.

What IS a Percent?

A *percent* (%) is a special ratio. It compares a number with 100.

What You NEED TO KNOW

A percent can be written as the ratio of the percent number to 100 or as its decimal equivalent. The decimal equivalent is determined by dividing by 100 or by simply moving the decimal point two places to the left.

Answers: **1.** 1 tab/0.4 mg or 0.4 mg/1 tab; **2.** 100 mg/1 mL or 1 mL/100 mg; **3.** 1 cap/450 mg or 450 mg/1 cap; **4.** 500 mg/0.7 mL or 0.7 mL/500 mg.

What You DO

EXAMPLE 1: Write 5% as a ratio and a decimal number.
To convert a percent to a ratio, place the number over 100 ($^5/_{100}$).

To convert a percent to its decimal equivalent, divide the percent by 100.

$$
\begin{array}{r}
0.05 \\
100\overline{)5.00} \\
\underline{5\ 00} \\
0
\end{array}
$$

Moving the decimal point two places to the left is a second method of converting a percent to its decimal equivalent (5% = 0.05). If no decimal is visible, place the decimal point at the right of the number (5 = 5.0).

EXAMPLE 2: 70% = 70/100 or 0.70 = 0.7 (Drop zeros at the right of the decimal numbers.)

EXAMPLE 3: $12^1/_2\% = \dfrac{12^1/_2}{100}$ or $100\,\overline{)12.5} = 0.125$

TAKE HOME POINTS

1. Place the percent number over 100 to change a percent to a ratio or fraction.
2. Move the decimal point two places to the left in the number to change a percent to its decimal equivalent.

Do You UNDERSTAND?

DIRECTIONS: Change each percent to a ratio and its decimal equivalent.

1. 10%
2. 8%
3. 1.5%
4. 0.05%
5. On page 24, circle the 12 ratios equal to those circled. Connect the equal ratios in the counting order of their numerators. Connect the last ratio to this first. What insect is formed?

11/12   11/4   11/15   15/30   11/20   1/6   1/5   1/8   3/2   3/6   3/4   3/5   3/7

1/18   1/16   1/14   1/12   1/10   1/4   (1/2)   1/3   1/7   1/9   1/11   1/13   1/15

14/28   2/1   ●   12/3   12/13   16/32   ☺   2/4   2/15   12/17   ●   12/18   4/8

3/9   3/10   3/11   3/12   3/13   3/14   3/15   11/13   11/14   11/16   11/17   11/18   11/19

4/5   10/9   10/11   (13/26)   4/9   4/3   10/5   10/3   10/40   (5/10)   10/4   4/6   4/10

2/7   3/8   4/7   5/18   6/15   8/13   10/7   9/4   11/33   12/25   1/24   7/24   8/14

12/24   8/4   6/18   ●   6/16   10/20   7/13   8/16   8/12   ●   8/18   6/13   6/12

7/6   7/7   7/5   7/42   7/35   7/28   (9/18)   7/15   7/16   7/2   7/49   7/3   7/21

9/10   5/4   5/15   11/22   5/12   5/13   9/14   5/14   9/12   7/14   9/11   5/3   9/5

What IS a Proportion?

A *proportion* is an equation of two ratios: $1:100 = 2:200$ or $^1/_{100} = {}^2/_{200}$.

What You NEED TO KNOW

The cross products are equal in a proportion. To determine the cross product, multiply the numerator of one fraction (ratio) by the denominator of the other fraction (ratio).

$$\frac{1}{100} = \frac{2}{200}$$
$$1 \times 200 = 2 \times 100$$
$$200 = 200$$

Determining the cross product will help you calculate medication doses. As with ratios, the units of measure and the value of numbers are used. Both ratios are set up to ensure that the same units of measure are in the same position. If carefully set up, a proportion is one of the safest ways to determine medication doses.

What You DO

EXAMPLE 1: **A dose of 10 mg is prescribed for your patient. You have the medication with a dose strength of 4 mg/1 mL. How much medication should you administer to your patient?**

To solve a proportion:
• Set up the first ratio (4 mg/1 mL). Include measurement units.
• Set up the second ratio with its units in the same position as the first ratio. Use an x for the missing part.

$$\frac{4 \text{ mg}}{1 \text{ mL}} = \frac{10 \text{ mg}}{x \text{ mL}}$$

• Cross multiply $4 \text{ mg} \times x \text{ mL} = 10 \text{ mg} \times 1 \text{ mL}$

• To determine the value of x, divide each side of the equation by the same number that is used to multiply x:

$$\underset{1}{\overset{1}{\frac{\cancel{4\ mg}}{\cancel{4\ mg}}}} \times x\ mL = \underset{1}{\overset{2.5}{\frac{\cancel{10\ mg}}{\cancel{4\ mg}}}} \times 1\ mL = 2.5\ mL$$

Answer: 2.5 mL

As a result of the previous calculation, administer 2.5 mL of medication. Remember, the accuracy of the answer can be confirmed by substituting the answer in place of the x in the original proportion and cross multiplying to solve the problem.

$$\frac{4}{1} = \frac{10}{2.5}$$
$$4 \times 2.5 = 10 \times 1$$
$$10 = 10$$

TAKE HOME POINTS

To solve a proportion:
1. Set up both ratios with the measurement units in the same position.
2. Determine the cross product by multiplying the numerator of the first fraction (ratio) by the denominator of the second fraction (ratio); place this answer (product) on one side of the equal sign. Multiply the denominator of the first fraction (ratio) by the numerator of the other fraction (ratio), and place this answer (product) on the other side of the equal sign.
3. Determine the value of x by dividing the number product by the quantity that multiplies x.

EXAMPLE 2: **You are asked to administer a dose of 200 mg. The available capsules are labeled 40 mg. How many capsules should be administered?**

$$\frac{40\ mg}{1\ capsule} = \frac{200\ mg}{x\ capsule}$$

$$40\ mg \times x\ capsule = 200\ mg \times 1\ capsule$$

$$x\ capsule = \underset{1}{\overset{5}{\frac{\cancel{200\ mg}}{\cancel{40\ mg}}}} \times 1\ capsule$$

Answer: $x = 5$ capsules

In both of these examples, the first ratio can be written in the reverse order. Instead of 40 mg/1 capsule, 1 capsule/40 mg can be used. However, the proportion should be written 1 capsule/40 mg = x capsule/200 mg; the result of the cross product is the same:

$$40\ mg \times x\ capsule = 200\ mg \times 1\ capsule$$

Do You UNDERSTAND?

DIRECTIONS: **Solve each proportion for *x*.**
1. 500 mg/3 mL = 350 mg/*x* mL
2. 0.3 mg/1 tablet = 0.75 mg/*x* tablets
3. 4 mg/2.6 mL = 5 mg/*x* mL
4. The order is for BuSpar 15 mg. You have BuSpar 5 mg tablets. How many tablets do you need?

References

Lumsden H, Doodson M: Neonatal drug calculations: a practical approach, *J Neonatal Nurs* 9(1):14-18, 2003.

Maag M: The effectiveness of an interactive multimedia learning tool on nursing students' math knowledge and self-efficacy, *CIN Comput Inform Nurs* 22(1): 26-33, 2004.

Tournaki N: The differential effects of teaching addition through strategy instruction versus drill and practice to students with and without learning disabilities, *J Learn Disabil* 36(5):449-58, 2003.

Wilson A: Nurses' math: researching a practical approach, *Nurs Standard* 17(47): 33-6, 2003.

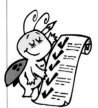

Notes

NCLEX® Review

You have reviewed mathematical concepts for calculating medication dosages. Now solve the following problems: Circle the correct answer.

1. You are to administer Gantrisin 1.5 g. The tablets you have are labeled Gantrisin 0.5 g. How many tablet(s) will you administer?
   1 1 tablet
   2 1½ tablets
   3 2 tablets
   4 3 tablets

2. How much atropine do you give a patient who weighs 250 lb if the order reads 0.3 mg for every 100 lb?
   1 8.3 mg
   2 83 mg
   3 7.5 mg
   4 0.75 mg

3. Morphine sulfate gr ⅙ is ordered. Your supply of morphine sulfate tablets is labeled gr ¼. How many tablet(s) will you use?
   1 1½ tablets
   2 1⅓ tablets
   3 1 tablet
   4 ⅔ tablet

4. Reglan (metoclopramide) 5 mg was ordered. You have available Reglan 10 mg/mL. Calculate the number of milliliters per dose.
   1 ⅕ mL/dose
   2 ½ mL/dose
   3 1 mL/dose
   4 1½ mL/dose

5. You are to administer penicillin 450,000 Units. The bottle of penicillin is labeled 300,000 Units/cc. How many cubic centimeters will you administer?
   1 0.4 cc
   2 0.8 cc
   3 2.5 cc
   4 1.5 cc

6. Short answer: What is the value of the "5" in the decimal 0.5 mL? _____

7. Short answer: If the total dose of the antibiotic cephalexin (Keflex) is 1000 mg/day and you have given 250 mg so far today to the patient, how many more milligrams are left to give the patient today? _____

8. Short answer: You are to administer two tablets each with the strength of 0.125 mg. What is the total dose? _____

9. True or False? A 1% solution is stronger (larger) than a 5% solution.

10. Short answer: You are asked to administer a 750 mg dose of the antibiotic ciproflaxin (Cipro). The available tablets are labeled 250 mg each. How many tablets should you administer?
    _____

NCLEX® Review Answers

1. **4** $0.5 \times 3 = 1.5$. The other three amounts are not enough.

2. **4** $0.3 \times 2.5 = 0.75$. 8.3 mg and 7.5 mg are too much. 83 mg is a lethal dose.

3. **4** $4 \times ⅙ = ⅔$. The other amounts are too much.

4. **2** $^5/_{10}$ = $^1/_2$. $^1/_5$ is not enough, and 1 and 1$^1/_2$ are too much.

5. **4** $^{450,000}/_{300,000}$ = 1.5. 0.4 cc is too small an amount, and 2.5 cc is too large. If you got 8 cc, you inverted the numerator and denominator.

6. tenths.

7. 1000 mg – 250 mg = 750 mg.

8. 0.25 mg.

9. False. $^5/_{100}$ is larger than $^1/_{100}$.

10. $^{250}/_1$ = $^{750}/_x$, so x = 3 tablets.

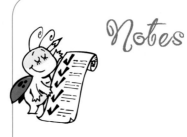

Notes

Systems of Measurement

What You WILL LEARN

After reading this chapter, you will know how to do the following:

✔ Define the metric, apothecary, and household measurement systems

✔ Interpret metric, household, and apothecary measurements

✔ Calculate and express international units and body surface area accurately

Medication dosages are measured in units. These units are categorized by either weight or volume. There are four systems of measurement you will use when calculating medication dosages: (1) the metric system; (2) the international unit system; (3) the household measurement or U.S. customary measurement system; and (4) the apothecary system. Medication dosages are usually given with abbreviations.

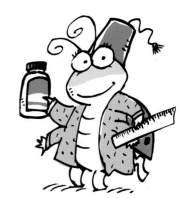

What IS the Metric System?

The *metric system* is a decimal system of weights and measurements based on the meter (m) as the unit of length, the gram (g) as the unit of weight, and the liter (L) as the unit of volume.

What You NEED TO KNOW

The metric system uses prefixes to indicate basic units. For the most part, you will be using only one larger measure, *kilo,* and two smaller measures, *milli* and *micro,* when calculating medication doses. However, the following table provides a full set of metric system prefixes.

Metric Units

Prefix (Symbol)	Power Times Standard Unit	Weight (Symbol)	Volume (Symbol)
Kilo (k)	10^3	Kilogram (kg)	
Hecto (h)	10^2	Hectogram (hg)	
Deka (dk)	10^1	Dekagram (dkg)	
Standard Unit	10^0	Gram (g)	Liter (L)
Deci (d)	10^{-1}	Decigram (dg)	Deciliter (dL)
Centi (c)	10^{-2}	Centigram (cg)	Centiliter (cL)
Milli (m)	10^{-3}	Milligram (mg)	Milliliter (mL)
Micro (mc)	10^{-6}	Microgram (mcg)	Microliter (mcL)
Nano (n)	10^{-9}	Nanogram (ng)	Nanoliter (nL)
Pico (p)	10^{-12}	Picogram (pg)	Picoliter (pL)

The following shows the relationship between the prefixes you will encounter when calculating medication doses:
- Kilogram (kg) = 1000 g
- Milligram (mg) = 1/1000 g
- 1 g = 1000 mg
- Microgram (mcg) = 1/1000 mg, or 1 mg = 1000 mcg

(Although you may see the µ symbol to represent "micro," JCAHO requires the use of "mc" or writing out the prefix "micro.")

Similarly, the volume measures you will use are:
- Milliliter (mL) = 1/1000 L, or 1000 mL = 1 L
- Microliter (mcL) = 1/1000 mL, or 1000 mcL = 1 mL

Sometimes cubic centimeter (cc) is used interchangeably with milliliter (mL).

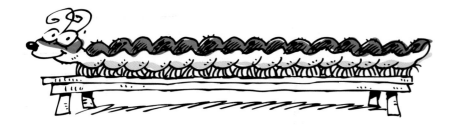

What You DO

When calculating medication doses, you will need to be able to convert kilo, standard, milli, and micro units of measure. Think of each unit as a floor in a building. The micro is the basement; the milli is the first floor; the standard unit is the second floor; and the kilo is the third floor or penthouse. To go from a larger unit to a smaller unit, you multiply by 1000 for each level descended; to go from a smaller to a larger unit, you divide by 1000 for each level ascended. Each floor descended or ascended requires you to move the decimal point three spaces. You can do the multiplication by moving the decimal point to the right and the division by moving the decimal point to the left.

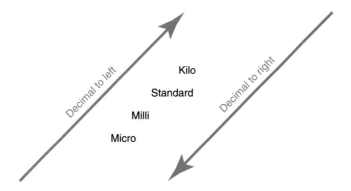

The following examples illustrate how to convert metric measurements.

EXAMPLE 1: **1.7 L =** _____ **mL**

To convert this measurement in the metric system you should:

• Decide whether you are converting the measurement from a smaller to a larger unit or vice versa (in this case, L to mL is a larger to smaller unit).

• Move decimal point 3 places to the right to go 1 floor down, L to mL (1.7 0 0 . mL).

Answer: 1.7 L is 1700 mL.

EXAMPLE 2: 0.01 mg = _____ g
This is a smaller to larger measurement unit, so you need to go one floor up by moving the decimal point 3 places to the left (. 0 0 0 . 01 mg).

Answer: 0.01 mg is 0.00001 g.

EXAMPLE 3: 200 mcg = _____ mg
This is a smaller to larger measurement unit, so you need to go one floor up by moving the decimal point 3 places to the left (. 2 0 0 . 00 mcg).

Answer: 200 mcg is 0.2 mg.

EXAMPLE 4: 0.5 cc = _____ mL

Answer: These are interchangeable units. Therefore 0.5 cc = 0.5 mL.

EXAMPLE 5: 250 cc = _____ L
This is a smaller to larger measurement unit, so you need to go one floor up by moving the decimal point 3 places to the left (. 2 5 0 .).

Answer: 250 cc is 0.25 L.

Do You UNDERSTAND?

DIRECTIONS: **Convert the following:**
1. 1.5 L = _____ mL
2. 2.5 cc = _____ L
3. 0.15 g = _____ mg
4. 5 mL = _____ cc
5. 2 kg = _____ g
6. 750 mcg = _____ mg

Answers: 1. 1500 mL; 2. 0.0025 L; 3. 150 mg; 4. 5 cc; 5. 2000 g; 6. 0.75 mg.

What IS an International Unit?

An *international unit* measures a drug in terms of its action or ability to produce a given result. It does not measure a drug in terms of its physical weight or volume. The term used to represent an international unit is Units. Heparin, insulin, and penicillin are just a few drugs that are measured in international units.

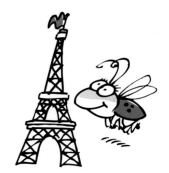

An international unit measures a drug in terms of its action or ability to produce a given result.

What You NEED TO KNOW

You will need to be able to recognize volume and dose strength listed on medication labels to prepare dosages for your patients.

What You DO

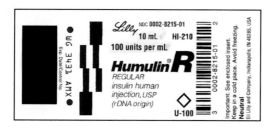

Humulin R insulin label. *Reproduced with permission of Eli Lilly and Co.*

EXAMPLE 1: Look at the above label and do the following:

• Determine the total volume of the vial.
  Answer: 10 mL

• Determine the dose strength.
  Answer: 100 Units/mL

• Prepare a dose of 10 Units.
  100 Units/1 mL = 10 Units/x mL
  100 Units $\times$ x mL = 10 Units $\times$ 1 mL

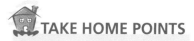

TAKE HOME POINTS

1. You must read labels carefully for volume and dose strength.
2. If necessary, review using proportion solving (Chapter 1)

$$\frac{\overset{1}{\cancel{100\ \text{Units}}}}{\underset{1}{\cancel{100\ \text{Units}}}} \times x\ \text{mL} = \frac{\overset{0.1}{\cancel{10\ \text{Units}}}}{\cancel{100\ \text{Units}}} \times 1\ \text{mL}$$

Answer: x mL = 0.1 mL. Therefore 0.1 mL is the correct dose.

Do You UNDERSTAND?

DIRECTIONS: **From the label below determine the following:**

1. The total volume of the vial.

   _____

2. The dose strength.

   _____

3. The preparation of a dose of 5000 Units.

   _____

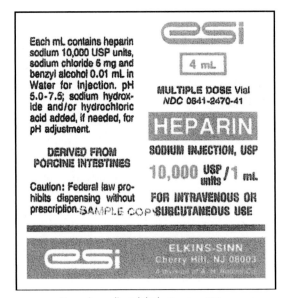

Heparin sodium label. *Courtesy Elkins-Sinn, a division of Baxter Health Care.*

What IS Body Weight?

Body weight is total weight that may include clothing that does not weigh more than 2 pounds. It is essential to determine an accurate weight by zeroing the scale before obtaining each patient's weight. Body weight is an important factor used to determine total drug doses for many life-saving medications. Body weight is usually measured in pounds (lb).

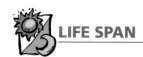

LIFE SPAN

Body weight is an important factor in calculating medication dosages, especially pediatric medications and chemotherapy.

What You NEED TO KNOW

Because many medications state doses in terms of kilograms, you will often need to convert pounds to kilograms. There are 2.2 pounds in 1 kilogram. Therefore to convert pounds to kilograms, divide the weight by 2.2 pounds.

What You DO

EXAMPLE 1: A child weighs 36 lb. What is her weight in kilograms?

To change pounds to kilograms you should:

- Divide the weight by 2.2 lb.

$$\frac{36}{2.2} = 16.36 \text{ kg}$$

- Round the weight to the nearest tenth.

    Answer: 36 lb = 16.4 kg

TAKE HOME POINTS

To convert pounds to kilograms:
1. Divide the weight in pounds by 2.2 lb.
2. Round the answer to the nearest tenth kilogram.

EXAMPLE 2: The prescribed reference dose for cefaclor (Ceclor) is 40 mg/kg. If your client weighs 24 lb, what dose should you administer?

$$\frac{24}{2.2} = 10.9 \text{ kg}$$

$$\frac{40 \text{ mg}}{1 \text{ kg}} = \frac{x \text{ mg}}{10.9 \text{ kg}}$$

Answer: The correct dosage is 436 mg.

Do You UNDERSTAND?

DIRECTIONS: Determine the following:

1. 100 lb = _____ kg
2. 63 lb = _____ kg
3. 12 lb = _____ kg
4. 37 lb = _____ kg
5. Cefixime (Suprax) is prescribed for a 14 lb infant. The reference dose for Suprax is 8 mg/kg. You have cefixime 100 mg/5 mL. Calculate the number of milliliter/dose for the infant.

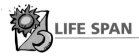

LIFE SPAN

BSA is an important factor in calculating doses for cancer chemotherapy and in pediatric medications.

What IS Body Surface Area?

Body surface area (BSA) is the measurement of the total skin area of a person in meters squared (m^2). You can calculate BSA using a person's weight and height.

What You NEED TO KNOW

- BSA can be determined by using a formula or a nomogram.
- If weight and height are in kilograms and centimeters, you would use the formula below to determine BSA:

$$BSA = \sqrt{\frac{weight\ (kg)\ \times\ height\ (cm)}{3600}}$$

- If weight and height are in pounds and inches, you would use the formula below to determine BSA:

$$BSA = \sqrt{\frac{weight\ (lb)\ \times\ height\ (in)}{3131}}$$

- The formulas used to determine BSA require the use of a calculator. If the units are kilograms and centimeters, use a calculator to multiply the weight × height (using correct units) and divide by 3600. If the units

Answers: 1. 45.5 kg; 2. 28.6 kg; 3. 5.5 kg; 4. 16.8 kg; 5. Use 2.6 mL.

are pounds and inches, multiply the weight × height and divide by 3131. Once you have that answer, use the $\sqrt{}$ key to determine BSA.

A nomogram is a calibrated scale that correlates heights (measured in centimeters or inches) and body weight (measured in pounds or kilograms) of adults and children. To use a nomogram to determine BSA:

- Take a straight edge (ruler) and very carefully locate the client's height and weight on the respective scales.
- Find your client's BSA at the point where the straight edge intersects the surface area (SA) scale.

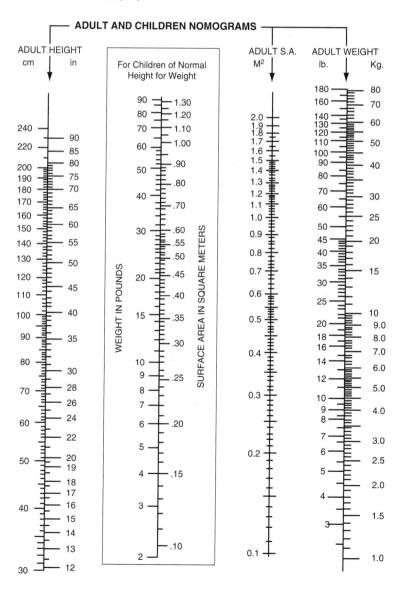

What You DO

EXAMPLE 1: **To determine the BSA of a person 56 inches tall and weighing 54 lb using a nomogram:**
- Place a straight edge (ruler) carefully on given height and weight.
  56 in = 54 1b
- Read SA scale.
  Answer: SA scale reads 1.0. Therefore BSA is 1.0 m².

EXAMPLE 2: **To determine BSA using a formula:**
- Multiply weight × height.
  54 lb × 56 in = 3024
- Because the measurements are in pounds and inches, divide by 3131 (you would divide by 3600 if the measurements were in kilograms and centimeters).
  3024 ÷ 3131 = 0.9658256
- Calculate the square root.
  $\sqrt{9658256} = 0.9827642$
- Round to the nearest tenth to determine BSA (see Chapter 1).
  9827642 = 1.0; the BSA is 1.0 m².

EXAMPLE 3: **Find the BSA of an adult who weighs 55 kg and measures 157.5 cm using a formula.**

$$\text{BSA} = \sqrt{\frac{55 \times 157.5}{3600}} = 1.55$$

Using this formula, the BSA would be 1.55 (the BSA would be 1.56 using a nomogram). In both cases you would round the answer to the nearest tenth, for a BSA of 1.6 m².

Do You UNDERSTAND?

DIRECTIONS: **Calculate the BSA in meters squared (m^2) for the following:**

1. A child whose weight is 60 lb and height 38 in.
2. An adult who weighs 68 kg and has a height of 160 cm.
3. A 4-year-old patient is 3 feet tall and weighs 53 lb. She receives an antineoplastic, antibiotic derivative on a weekly basis. The order is for 20 mg/m^2 per dose. The 4-year-old's dose in milligram/dose is:
   a. 20 mg/dose
   b. 16.0 mg/dose
   c. 1800 mg/dose

What IS Household Measurement?

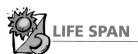

LIFE SPAN

Household measurement, also referred to as *U.S. Customary Measurement,* may appear familiar to you because it is used in cookbooks and in recipes.

Household measurement is used in medication doses for children and those being cared for at home.

What You NEED TO KNOW

The household units that you will most commonly use when working with medication doses are:

- Drop, abbreviated gtt.
- Teaspoon, abbreviated t or tsp = 60 gtt = 5 mL (see table of U.S. Customary System of Volume Measurements).
- Tablespoon, abbreviated T or tbsp = 15 mL (see table of Equivalents for U.S. Customary and Metric Measure).

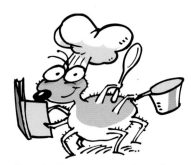

Household measurement is used in cookbooks and in recipes.

U.S. Customary System of Volume Measurement

4 quarts (qt)	=	1 gallon (gal)
2 pints (pt)	=	1 quart (qt)
2 measuring cups (c)	=	1 pint (pt)
8 fluid ounces (fl oz)	=	1 measuring cup
2 tablespoons (T or tbsp)	=	1 fluid ounce (fl oz)
3 teaspoons (tsp)	=	1 tablespoon (tbsp)
1 teaspoon (tsp)	=	.1 fluid dram (fl dr)
1 drop (gtt)	=	1 minim (m)
4 microdrops (µgtt)	=	1 drop (gtt)

Equivalents for U.S. Customary and Metric Measure

U.S. Customary Measure	Metric Weight Measure
2.2 lb	1 kg
2 tbsp	30 g
0.353 oz	1 g
15-16 gr	1 g
1 gr	60-65 mg
	Metric Volume Measure
1 gal	3785 mL
1 qt	960-1000 mL
1 pt	480-500 mL
1 c	240-250 mL
1 fl oz = 2 T or tbsp	30-32 mL
1 tbsp = 4 fl dr	15-16 mL
1 tsp = 1 fl dr	4-5 mL
60 µgtt	1 mL
15-16 gtt = 15-16 m	1 mL
1 gtt = 1 m	0.06-0.07 mL

What You DO

EXAMPLE 1: 2.5 T = ____ mL

When working with medication dosages, you must:

- Recognize abbreviations and symbols, such as tbsp or T for tablespoon.
- Know conversion factors.
- Be able to make calculations using proportions or have conversion tables available.
- Because 1 T = 15 mL, you would use the following proportion:

$$\frac{15 \text{ mL}}{1 \text{ T}} = \frac{x \text{ mL}}{2.5 \text{ T}}$$

- Convert the dose in the following way:

$$\frac{15\ \text{mL} \times 2.5\ \text{T}}{1\ \text{T}} = x\ \text{mL}$$

37.5 mL = x mL

Answer: 2.5 T = 37.5 mL

EXAMPLE 2: 3 tsp = _____ mL

- Because 1 tsp = 4 to 5 mL, you would convert the dose in the following way:

$$\frac{5\ \text{mL}}{1\ \text{tsp}} = \frac{x\ \text{mL}}{3\ \text{tsp}}$$

15 mL = x mL

Answer: 3 tsp = 15 mL

EXAMPLE 3: 20 mL = _____ tsp

- Because 4 to 5 mL = 1 tsp, you would convert the dosage in the following way:

$$\frac{1\ \text{tsp}}{5\ \text{mL}} = \frac{x\ \text{tsp}}{20\ \text{mL}}$$

Answer: 20 mL = 4 tsp

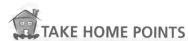

TAKE HOME POINTS

When using household measurements, remember that:
1. 1 drop = 1 gtt.
2. 60 gtt = 1 teaspoon (tsp or t) = 5 mL.
3. 1 tablespoon (T or tbsp) = 15 mL.
4. You should always have conversion tables available.

Do You UNDERSTAND?

DIRECTIONS: **Determine the following:**

1. 2.5 tsp = _____ mL
2. 45 mL = _____ T
3. 10 mL = _____ tsp
4. A child's medication dosage reads 120 gtt once a week. How many teaspoons should the child be given weekly?
5. The dosage protocol for giving Tylenol elixir (elix) is 1 gr/yr PO q4hr prn. Your patient, Audra, is 24 months old, and you have been asked to administer Children's Tylenol elix 160 mg/tsp. Calculate the number of teaspoons per dose, and color the appropriate number of spoons.

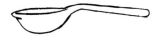
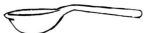
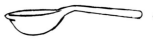
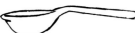

Answers: 1. 12.5 mL; 2. 3 T; 3. 2 tsp; 4. 2 tsp; 5. ³⁄₈ tsp.

What IS Apothecary Measurement?

Apothecary measurement is one of the oldest drug measurement systems. Although it is infrequently used, it is still seen on drug labels and prescriptions. Therefore it is important for you to understand this system to administer medications safely.

What You NEED TO KNOW

The apothecary system uses fractions ($\frac{1}{2}$, $2\frac{3}{4}$), rather than decimals (0.5, 2.75). For larger quantities, Roman numerals (with dots over the *I*s to avoid confusion) are sometimes used. For example:

$$1 = \dot{I}, 2 = \ddot{II}, 3 = \dddot{III}, 4 = \dot{I}V, 5 = V, 6 = V\dot{I}, 7 = V\ddot{II},$$
$$8 = V\dddot{III}, 9 = \dot{I}X, 10 = X.$$

The symbol *ss* is sometimes used for $\frac{1}{2}$.

For example, XXss = $20\frac{1}{2}$, $V\dddot{III}$ss = $8\frac{1}{2}$.

In the apothecary system, the unit measure comes before the numerical quantity.

The basic weight measure is the grain, abbreviated gr, and gr 1 = 60 mg.

In the apothecary system, volume is indicated as follows:

- Minim, abbreviated m or min = 1 drop
- Dram, abbreviated dr or ʒ = 60 min = 5 mL
- Ounce, abbreviated oz or ℥ = 30 mL

What You DO

EXAMPLE 1: **Express 5 minims in correct form.**

In the apothecary system, you need to:

- Know symbols *min* or *m* for minim.
- Place symbol first and use either Roman or Arabic numbers.

Answer: m V or m 5, or min V or min 5

EXAMPLE 2: **Express one-quarter grain in correct form.**

Answer: gr $\frac{1}{4}$

EXAMPLE 3: **Express 4 drams in correct form.**
Answer: dr 4 or dr İV, or ʒ 4 or ʒ İV

EXAMPLE 4: **Determine the following:**
gr $^1/_6$ = ___ mg
Because gr 1 = 60 mg, you would convert the dosage in the following way:

$$\frac{60 \text{ mg}}{\text{gr } 1} = \frac{x \text{ mg}}{\text{gr } ^1/_6}$$

Answer: 10 mg = x mg. Therefore gr $^1/_6$ = 10 mg (refer to Chapter 1 for solving).

EXAMPLE 5: **Determine the following:**
60 mL = ___ oz
Because 1 oz = 30 mL, you would convert the dosage in the following way:

$$\frac{1 \text{ oz}}{30 \text{ mL}} = \frac{x \text{ oz}}{60 \text{ mL}}$$

Answer: 2 oz = x oz. Therefore 60 mL = 2 oz.

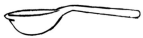**TAKE HOME POINTS**

When working with the apothecary system, remember:
1. Measurement units are written before the number.
2. Weight measures, grain (gr) = 60 mg.
3. Volume measures:
   minim (min) = 1 drop
   dram (dr or ʒ) = min 60 = 5 mL
   ounce (oz or ʒ) = 30 mL
4. Have conversion tables available.

Do You UNDERSTAND?

DIRECTIONS: **Determine the following:**
1. gr 6$^1/_2$ = _____ mg
2. $^1/_2$ oz = _____ mL
3. 600 mg = gr _____
4. gr $^1/_{300}$ = _____ mg
5. Michael is 36 months old and needs children's acetaminophen elixir (180 mg/tsp) immediately. The dosage should be gr 1 per year orally. Calculate the number of teaspoons/dose that Michael should receive. Then color in the dosage in the spoons below.

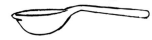 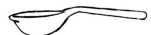 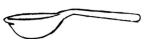 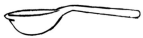

Answers: 1. 390 mg; 2. 15 mL; 3. gr 10; 4. 0.2 mg; 5. 1 tsp.

References

Hutton M: Calculations for new prescribers, *Nurs Standard* 17(25):42-52, 2003.

McCaffery M: Pain control. Switching from IV to PO: maintaining pain relief in the transition, *AJN* 103(5):62-3, 2003.

Roberts WC: Measuring the meter and using the metric system, *Am J Cardiol* 91(7):922-3, 2003.

VanGijn J: The human measure, (Dutch), *Nederlands Tijdschrif voor Geneeskunde* 148(1):1-3, 2004.

Waldrop JB: Advisor forum. Calculating complex conversions—made easy! *Clinical Advisor* 5(4):82, 2002.

NCLEX® Review

Solve these "real life" situations.
Circle the correct answer.

1. A physician prescribes digoxin 0.15 mg intravenous slow push (IVSP) for one of your patients. You have digoxin 0.5 mg/2 mL in stock. Calculate the number of milliliters per dose that your patient should have.
   1 6 mL/dose
   2 0.6 mL/dose
   3 600 mL/dose
   4 15 mL/dose

2. Calcium gluconate comes in a vial of 1 g/10 mL. The prescription indicates that you should give the patient 320 mg of calcium gluconate IVSP. Calculate the number of milliliters per dose that your patient should have.
   1 3.2 mL/dose
   2 0.032 mL/dose
   3 320 mL/dose
   4 3200 mL/dose

3. Adriamycin (doxorubicin HCL) 20 mg/m² is the prescribed chemotherapy for Mrs. Cortez, who is 57 inches tall and weighs 142 pounds. You are double checking the dosage the pharmacy sent you (Adriamycin 34 mg in 50 cc of D_5W). The nomogram indicates that Mrs. Cortez's body surface area (BSA) is 1.7 m². Did you receive the correct dosage from the pharmacy?
   1 Yes
   2 No
   3 It is not possible to determine dosage from the information given.
   4 Chemotherapy is not prescribed by BSA.

4. If Mrs. Cortez, still 57 inches tall, returns at a later time weighing 200 pounds, will her dose be the same?

1 Yes
2 No
3 It is not possible to determine dosage from the information given.
4 Chemotherapy is not prescribed by BSA.

5. Maritzah is 9 years old and weighs 67.5 lb. The prescribed dose for erythromycin stearate is 20 mg/kg qid. You have erythromycin stearate 200 mg/5 mL in stock. Calculate the number of teaspoons of erythromycin per dose for Maritzah.
   1 3 tsp/dose
   2 1 tsp/dose
   3 3/4 tsp/dose
   4 4 tsp/dose

6. Bill, a 15 year-old boy, weighs 98 lb and is to receive an initial insulin dose for hyperglycemia and ketonuria. The prescription reads, "regular insulin 0.1 Units/kg SQ qid." How many units of regular insulin will Bill receive at each dose?
   1 9.8 Units/dose
   2 4.5 Units/dose
   3 45 Units/dose
   4 98 Units/dose

7. Short answer: You are to administer 2 g of a certain medication within 24 hours. Each tablet is 500 mg. How many tablets should you give in 24 hours? _____

8. Short answer: You are to administer 1 L of normal saline (NS), intravenously, over 24 hours. You have on hand 250 mL bags of NS. How many bags of NS should you hang in 24 hours? _____

9. Short answer: Heparin sodium injection comes in 10,000 Units/mL. You are to administer 5,000 Units. Your nurse colleague says you should

administer 2 mL of heparin sodium. Is your nurse colleague correct? _____

10. Short answer: You are to administer to your patient 15 mL of liquid Colace as a stool softener. You draw up 0.5 oz of Colace liquid. Is this correct? _____

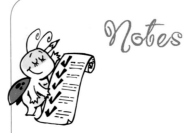

NCLEX® Review Answers

1. **2** 0.5 mg × x = 2 mL × 0.15, so x = 0.6. If you go 6 mL, you forgot the decimal point. 15 mL is too much, and 600 mL is a lethal dose.

2. **1** 1000:10 = 320:x, or $^{3200}/_{1000}$ = 3.2. If you got 0.032, 320, or 3200, you converted grams to milligrams incorrectly.

3. **1** Yes. 1.7 × 20 = 34. You need BSA and prescription to calculate the answer, and chemotherapy is prescribed by BSA.

4. **2** No. Dosage is based on BSA, which is based on weight. Chemotherapy is prescribed by BSA, and changes in weight do affect the dosage of chemotherapy.

5. **1** 67.5 ÷ 2.2 = 30.68 × 20 = 614 mg rounded = 15 mL ÷ 5 mL = 3 tsp/dose.

6. **2** (9.8 ÷ 2.2) × 0.1 = 4.5. 9.8 Units/dose is too much; consider Units/kg. 45 Units/dose and 98 Units/dose are overdoses.

7. 1 g = 1000 mg, so 4 tablets of 500 mg each.

8. 1 L = 1000 mL, so 4 bags of 250 mL NS each.

9. No, you should administer 0.5 mL.

10. Yes, 1 oz = 30 mL.

Temperature Conversion

What You WILL LEARN

After reading this chapter, you will know how to do the following:

✔ Name two different types of temperature scales.
✔ Convert between Fahrenheit and Celsius temperatures.
✔ Convert between Celsius and Fahrenheit temperatures.

Reading and recording a patient's body temperature is an important step in assessing his or her need for medication or emergency care. It is also a valuable tool for preventing negative health outcomes, such as minor infections that turn into sepsis. There are two scales used to measure temperature: the *Fahrenheit* (F) *scale* and the *Celsius* (C) or *centigrade scale.* Although you can use Celsius-Fahrenheit equivalency tables to convert temperatures, you should also be able to make these conversions using simple formulas.

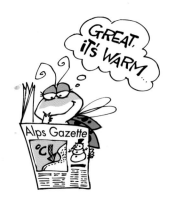

What IS Fahrenheit to Celsius?

The formula for converting from the Fahrenheit scale to the Celsius scale is

$$C = \frac{5}{9}(F - 32)$$

What You NEED TO KNOW

To convert a given temperature from Fahrenheit to Celsius:
* Subtract 32 from the temperature.
* Multiply by $\frac{5}{9}$ or, if you prefer, divide by 1.8.

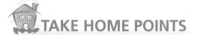

TAKE HOME POINTS

To convert a temperature from Fahrenheit to Celsius:
1. Subtract 32 from the Fahrenheit temperature.
2. Divide by 1.8 OR multiply by $\frac{5}{9}$.
3. Round to the nearest tenth.

What You DO

EXAMPLE 1: Convert 98.6° F to Celsius.

To find the answer:
* Subtract 32 from the temperature.

$$
\begin{array}{r}
98.6 \\
-\,32.0 \\
\hline
66.6
\end{array}
$$

* Multiply by $\frac{5}{9}$.

$$\frac{5}{\cancel{9}_1} \times \frac{\overset{7.4}{\cancel{66.6}}}{1} = \frac{5}{1} \times \frac{7.4}{1} = 37$$

OR

* Divide by 1.8.

66.6 ÷ 1.8 = 37

Therefore 98.6° F = 37° C

Fill in the Celsius equivalent to 98.6° F on the thermometer below:

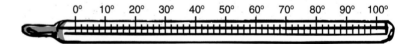

EXAMPLE 2: 102° F = _____ ° C

102 − 32 = 70 and $\frac{5}{9} \times 70$ (or 70 ÷ 1.8) = 38.88

If you round your answer to the nearest tenth, 102° F = 38.9° C.

Do You UNDERSTAND?

DIRECTIONS: **Convert each Fahrenheit temperature to Celsius.**

1. 96° F _____ C
2. 101.5° F _____ C
3. 104° F _____ C
4. Water boils at 212° F. At what temperature Celsius does water boil?
   _____ C

What IS Celsius to Fahrenheit?

The formula for converting from the Celsius scale to the Fahrenheit scale is

   $F = \frac{9}{5} C + 32$.

What You NEED TO KNOW

To convert a given temperature from Celsius to Fahrenheit:

- Multiply the given temperature by $\frac{9}{5}$ or 1.8.
- Add 32 to the product (the answer when you multiply).

What You DO

EXAMPLE 1: **Convert 35° C to Fahrenheit.**

To find the answer:

- Multiply the temperature by $\frac{9}{5}$ or 1.8.

$$\frac{\overset{7}{\cancel{35}}}{1} \times \frac{9}{\underset{1}{\cancel{5}}} = \frac{7}{1} \times \frac{9}{1} = 63$$

OR

$$\begin{array}{r} 35 \\ \times\ 1.8 \\ \hline 280 \\ 35\ \ \\ \hline 63.0 \end{array}$$

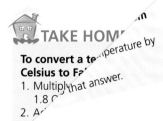

TAKE HOM
...on
To convert a te...perature by
Celsius to Fa'
1. Multiply that answer.
   1.8 C
2. A'

• Add 32 to the product.
63 + 32 = 95
Therefore 35° C = 95° F

EXAMPLE 2: **39° C = _____° F**
39 × 1.8 = 70.2 + 32 = 102.2
Therefore 39° C = 102.2° F

Do You UNDERSTAND?

DIRECTIONS: Convert each Celsius temperature to Fahrenheit.

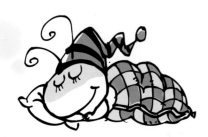

1. 36° C _____ F
2. 37° C _____ F
3. 41° C _____ F
4. Leo is planning to go on a camping trip this weekend. His sleeping bag is guaranteed to keep him warm in temperatures no lower than 10° below 0° F. The local news has reported that the overnight low temperature will be 18° C. Will Leo's sleeping bag be enough to keep him warm? What will the overnight low temperature be in degrees Fahrenheit?
   _____ F

Temperature Equivalency Table

	Scale	
	Fahrenheit (F)	Celsius (C)
Boiling point of water	212°	100°
Normal human body temperature	98.6°	37°
Freezing point of water	32°	0°

References

Conversion of units, www.chemie.fu-berlin.de/chemistry/general/units_en.html
Weather, www.usatoday.com/weather/wtempcf.htm

Answers: 1. 96.8° F; 2. 98.6° F; 3. 105.8° F; 4. The sleeping bag is enough, 64.4° F.

NCLEX® Review

Circle the correct answer.

1. Mrs. Krazniak is to begin triple antibiotic therapy if her temperature reaches, or goes higher than, 102° F. Your hospital only has thermometers that indicate temperature in Celsius. At what Celsius temperature would you begin Mrs. Krazniak's antibiotic therapy?
   1 74.4° C
   2 38.9° C
   3 56.7° C
   4 24.7° C

2. Mr. Popovsky can be transferred from the recovery room to his regular hospital room when his body temperature reaches 98° F. You only have a Celsius thermometer. What must Mr. Popovsky's temperature be in degrees Celsius so that he can be transferred to his regular room?
   1 36.7° C
   2 72.7° C
   3 54.4° C
   4 22.4° C

3. Molly McCarthy is to be placed on a hypothermia blanket when her temperature is equal to or greater than 39° C. You have only a Fahrenheit thermometer. At what degree Fahrenheit would you first place Molly on the hypothermia blanket?
   1 71° F
   2 39.5° F
   3 102.2° F
   4 127.8° F

4. Six-year-old Michael Woods has a history of ear infections. His parents have been instructed by the physician to begin antibiotic therapy if Michael's temperature is above 38.2° C. However, Michael's parents only have an ear (tympanic) thermometer that displays results in degrees Fahrenheit. At what temperature, in degrees Fahrenheit, should they begin antibiotic therapy for Michael?
   1 126.3° F
   2 68.8° F
   3 100.8° F
   4 91.8° F

5. True or False? The normal body temperature of an adult human is 37° C.

6. Fill in the blank: A temperature of 37° C is equal to _____ ° F.

7. Short answer: You are to call the physician if your patient's oral temperature exceeds 101° F. Your patient's oral temperature is 39° C. Do you call the physician? _____

8. Short answer: "Administer 650 mg acetaminophen (Tylenol) orally for temperature greater than 38.6° C" is prescribed. Your patient's temperature is 100.2° F. Do you administer the Tylenol? _____
_____

9. Short answer: Prescription for your patient reads "Use hyperthermia blanket if rectal temperature is less than 35.6° C." Your patient's rectal temperature is 95.7° F. Do you use the hyperthermia blanket? _____

10. True or False? Your patient's rectal temperature is 41° C. You know that the human brain can initiate seizures at temperatures greater than 105° F. Therefore you should initiate measures to decrease this patient's temperature to help prevent seizures.
_____

NCLEX® Review Answers

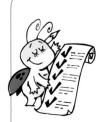

Notes

1. **2** 102 − 32 = 70; 70 ÷ 1.8 = 38.9. 74.4 is incorrect; you need to subtract 32, not add 32. If you got 56.7 or 24.7, you need to subtract 32 first, then divide by 1.8.

2. **1** 98 − 32 = 66; 66 ÷ 1.8 = 36.7° C. 72.7° C is incorrect; you need to subtract 32, not add 32. 54.4° C and 22.4° C are also incorrect; you need to subtract 32 first, then divide by 1.8.

3. **3** 32 × 1.8 = 70.2; 70.2 + 32 = 102.2° F. 71° F and 127.8° F are incorrect; you must multiply by 1.8 first, then add 32. 39.5° F is also incorrect; you used the wrong formula for conversion.

4. **3** 38.2 × 1.8 = 68.76; 68.76 ÷ 32 = 100.76 = 100.8° F (when rounded). 126.3° F and 68.8° F are incorrect; you need to multiply first by 1.8, then add 32. 91.8° F is also incorrect; after you multiplied 38.2 by 1.8, you need to add 32, not 23.

5. True.

6. 98.6.

7. Yes, 39° C = 102.2° F.

8. No, 38.6° C = 101.5° F.

9. Yes, 35.6° C = 96° F.

10. True. 41° C = 105.8° F.

General Principles of Medication Administration

What You WILL LEARN

After reading this chapter, you will know how to do the following:

✔ Identify required parts of a valid prescription and medication label for use in the clinical setting.

✔ Describe the nurses' legal responsibilities in administering medications.

✔ Recognize safety measures for appropriate administration of medications.

As a health care provider, one of your most important responsibilities is the administration of medications to your patients. Despite any error made in the prescription or delivery of a medication by a prescriber or pharmacy, the provider who administers that medication is legally and ethically responsible for any negative consequences to the patient. Although health care providers and pharmacists work together to promote the safe and effective use of prescription medications, it is the provider who is most likely to monitor their effects on patients. For these reasons, you must know the appropriate medications for the patient's condition, maximum and minimum drug dosage, contraindications, actions, and side effects for each medication that you administer.

What IS a Valid Prescription?

In a health care facility, written medication prescriptions or orders are given using a prescription or order sheet containing the patient's full name as stated on the patient's chart. A prescription includes the following information:

- Date it was written
- Brand or generic name of the drug
- Amount of the medication to be given
- Route of administration
- Frequency the medication is to be taken
- Special instructions
- Signature of a licensed provider (for the prescription to be legally valid)

Teresa Currant
Medcenter Drive
Northbrook, AR 91988
(555) 123-4321

Name _Joseph Smith_   Age _36_

Address _1520 High St_   Date _10/3/05_

Rx _Keflex 500 mgm by mouth Three times a day_

Label _✓_

Safety cap _✓_

Refill _2_ times   _____ MD

What You NEED TO KNOW

If the medication is to be "given as needed" (indicated by the abbreviation *prn*), the purpose for which the medication is being prescribed should also be included in the written order, such as for pain. An order is in effect for a specified amount of time, until a certain amount of the medication is given to the patient, or the order is changed or discontinued.

In certain situations or emergencies, you may need to take orders verbally (in person or by telephone) and write them on the order sheet in a patient's chart. When obtaining verbal prescription orders, you must request the same information required for written prescription orders. You should also verify the prescription order with the prescriber by repeating it as you have recorded it on the patient's order sheet. Write the prescriber's name, the fact that the prescription order has been made in person or by telephone, and sign the order. Finally, request that the prescriber sign verbal prescription orders within the time frame specified by the facility.

To determine the correct time for your patient to receive a prescribed medication, you must consider the purpose for which medicine is being given, the absorption rate of the medication, the potential interactions that it may have with other medications or with food, and the possible side effects that the medication may cause. Although prescription orders usually include guidelines to help you do this, these guidelines may vary widely. Fortunately, most health care facilities have routine times for administering medications (planned in conjunction with stated times for meals). Because these times differ from facility to facility, you will need to be familiar with your facility's medication-administration schedule.

To enhance safety and prevent errors in the administration of medication to patients, many facilities are now converting to the use of 24-hour, or military, time. This technique for telling time uses four digits to indicate hours and minutes; the first two digits represent the hours, and the last two digits represent the minutes. For example, midnight is expressed as 0000 hours, 1 AM as 0100 hours, 2 AM as 0200 hours, and so on. Afternoon times can be quickly computed in military time by adding 12 to the PM time. For example, noon is expressed as 1200 hours, so 6:00 PM would be converted by adding 12 + 6 = 1800 hours.

As a health care provider, you must also correctly interpret written and verbal medication orders. To do this safely, it is now recommended that prescriptions be written out and that abbreviations not be used. Since abbreviations may still be used, it is important to be familiar with them. Abbreviations can be written using uppercase or lowercase letters, depending on facility policy or regional practice. Common abbreviations related to route of medication delivery are summarized in the following table.

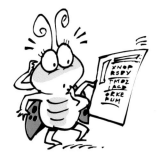

Abbreviation	Term	Definition
PO	Orally	By mouth
SL	Sublingually	Under the tongue
ID	Intradermally	Injection into the dermis, just below the epidermal layer of skin
SubQ, SC, or SQ	Subcutaneously	Injection into tissue just below the dermal layer of the skin
IM	Intramuscularly	Injection into a muscle
IV	Intravenously	Injection into a vein
IVSP	Intravenous slow push	Injected slowly into a peripheral venous access port closest to the intravenous catheter
IVPB	Intravenous piggyback	Administered by a secondary IV fluid system attached to the primary IV system
TD	Transdermally	Applied to the skin by a patch

Lowercase Roman numerals often used in writing medication orders include the following:

Symbol	Meaning
i	One
ii	Two
iii	Three
iv	Four
ss	One half

Common scheduling abbreviations used in giving medications include the following:

ac	Before meals
pc	After meals
hs	At bedtime
qd	Every day
bid	Twice a day
tid	Three times a day
qid	Four times a day
qh	Every hour
q2h	Every 2 hours
q4h	Every 4 hours
q8h	Every 8 hours
q12h	Every 12 hours
qod	Every other day
prn	As needed
stat	Immediately

Currently, most medications are obtained in individual or unit doses from the pharmacy or the patient care unit. Most are packaged in the required dose and are ready for administration. However, if the medication is not available in the required strength, or the medication is ordered in one system of measurement and available in another, you will need to calculate the correct dose of the medication.

TAKE HOME POINTS

1. For a prescription to be legally valid, it must be signed by the prescriber.
2. The health care provider must correctly interpret written and verbal medication orders.

What You DO

Doses of medications with a narrow safety margin, such as digoxin, heparin, or insulin, must be verified by another health care provider before you administer the medication to your patient. This is because receiving these medications in error or errors in dose or medication selection could have immediate, life-threatening consequences for your patient.

If you need to calculate the correct dose of a medication, remember to double check your results (using a calculator, if possible). Errors in dose or medication selection could have immediate, life-threatening consequences for your patient.

Do You UNDERSTAND?

DIRECTIONS: **Write the abbreviations for the following terms:**

1. Intravenous slow push   _____
2. Transdermally   _____
3. Subcutaneously   _____ or _____, _____
4. Intramuscularly   _____
5. Intravenously   _____
6. Intravenously piggyback   _____
7. Sublingually   _____
8. By mouth   _____

DIRECTIONS: **State the following times in military time:**

9. 8 AM   _____
10. 10 AM   _____
11. 2 PM   _____

12. 6 PM   _____
13. 10:30 PM   _____
14. Midnight   _____

DIRECTIONS: **Write the abbreviations for the following:**

15. Three times a day   _____
16. Every hour   _____
17. Every other day   _____
18. Twice a day   _____
19. After meals   _____
20. At bedtime   _____
21. Immediately   _____
22. As needed   _____
23. Four times a day   _____
24. Once a day   _____
25. Every 4 hours   _____
26. Before meals   _____

What IS a Drug Label?

A *drug label* is a label placed on each drug container that has certain iden-tifying information. Information on a drug label includes the medica-tion's generic, trade, and/or chemical names; form (tablet, suspension, etc.); strength; expiration date; manufacturer; lot number; recommended storage; and other important information.

What You NEED TO KNOW

The drug label identifies the medication's trade name and generic name (registered by manufacturer), and route of administration. With oral route of administration, medications are either in solid form (tablets, scored tablets, chewable sublingual tablets, enteric coated tablets [dissolved in the intestine], timed-release tablets, capsules, time-released capsules, gelatin capsules, powders) or liquid form (elixirs, solutions, suspensions). Parenteral (administered through injection) medications come as liquids or powders. The label also includes the drug strength (amount of drug that is available in a specific unit of measure, such as milligrams/capsule or milligrams/milliliters), expiration date (date after which the drug potency is compromised and the drug should not be dispensed), storage information (room temperature or refrigeration), lot number (refers to a batch of drugs that were manufactured at a specific time; is used if a medication recall is required), National Drug Code (NDC) a drug-specific number required by the federal government, and bar code (electronic system used with tracking, ordering, charging, and in some settings to compare a drug with a specific patient).

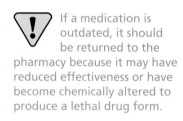

If a medication is outdated, it should be returned to the pharmacy because it may have reduced effectiveness or have become chemically altered to produce a lethal drug form.

What You DO

You must read each drug label carefully and compare it to the prescription to ensure that you are administering the correct drug in the correct dose. You must also check to see that the drug has been stored correctly and that it has not surpassed its expiration date. If a drug is outdated, it should be returned to the pharmacy because it may have reduced effectiveness or have become chemically altered.

TAKE HOME POINTS

1. Carefully read the medication name on the label three times to ensure accuracy in administering the correct medication. Many medications have similar names with minor spelling variations.
2. Read the medication strength on the label three times to ensure accuracy in administering the correct dose.

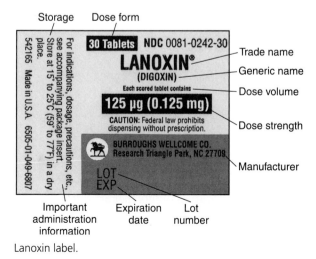

Lanoxin label.

Do You UNDERSTAND?

DIRECTIONS: **Label each statement *True* or *False*.**

1. _____ The drug form is typically listed on the drug labels.
2. _____ A drug label typically contains a list of adverse effects that may be caused by the medication.

What IS the Nurse's Legal Responsibility in Medication Administration?

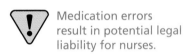

Medication errors result in potential legal liability for nurses.

Legally, nurses are required to administer medication as prescribed by the licensed health care provider (either a physician or advanced practice nurse). As nurse, you are responsible for your own actions and are professionally accountable for accuracy and precision when administering medication.

Nurses are guided by the *American Nurses' Association Standards of Nursing Practice,* their home state's *Nurse Practice Act,* and their local state board of nursing's *Rules and Regulations.* Because laws governing medication administration vary from state to state, nurses who move to new locations should investigate these laws before beginning work in a new location.

There are many reliable sources of drug information. Resources that are developed to ensure drug uniformity and are recognized as reliable include:

- *The United States Pharmacopeia (USP)* www.usp.org
- *The British Pharmacopeia* www.pharmacopoeia.org.uk
- *British National Formulary (BNF)* http://bnf.vhn.net

What You NEED TO KNOW

A medication error may result in a patient receiving the wrong medication or dose. Examples of incorrect practice leading to errors include the following:

- Lack of familiarity with an ordered medication.
- Lack of communication in verbal or written medication orders.
- Failure to question medication orders that are unclear.
- Failure to adhere to established procedures in administering medications.

Answers: 1. **True;** 2. **False.**

- Failure to recognize adverse drug reactions.
- Faulty dose calculation.

To prevent errors, you need to be familiar with the medication being administered by having certain drug information, such as the drug classification, action, appropriate route and dosage, adverse effects, and any nursing responsibilities unique to the specific medication.

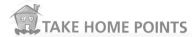

TAKE HOME POINTS

1. Always seek medication information from a reliable source (before administering any medication) when you feel that your knowledge of a particular drug is incomplete.
2. Always question any unreasonable medication order.

What You DO

If any portion of the medication order seems unreasonable or incorrect, it is your duty to question the prescription and seek clarification before administering the medication. If the prescriber refuses to clarify, is unavailable for clarification, or upholds an unreasonable medication order that is inconsistent with acceptable medication guidelines (e.g., normal dose range), you should seek suitable subsequent action from a supervisor. In addition, you must document the situation following the guidelines of your medical facility.

Do You UNDERSTAND?

DIRECTIONS: **Label each statement *True* or *False*.**

1. _____ The physician is responsible for the accuracy of all medication orders. If an unreasonable order is written and you know that the dosage is outside the normal range, you should legally disregard the order and not administer the medication.

2. _____ If you are unaware of the action of a prescribed medication, you should seek that specific information before administering the medication.

3. _____ If a drug label is outdated, you should return it to the pharmacy.

Answers: 1. **False**, 2. **True**, 3. **True**.

What IS a Safety Measure in Medication Administration?

In addition to the legal measures mentioned previously, safe and accurate administration of medication requires that you follow safe procedures in the administration of medications. Several guidelines have been devised to ensure safety.

What You NEED TO KNOW

As a health care provider administering medications, you need to be aware of the Six Rights of Medication Administration. The six rights promote assurance that the medication administered is the right drug, in the right dose, that it is given to the right patient, at the right time, in the right route, and has the right (correct) documentation. As stated earlier, when working with medications you also need to be aware of safe handling and storage procedures. To maintain drug stability, it may be necessary to control elements, such as temperature, moisture, and light. You should always check the expiration date to ensure drug strength and desired action.

What You DO

There are several steps you should take before administering medication. These include checking to see if the patient is allergic to any medications to prevent an adverse drug reaction. In addition, you should always wash your hands thoroughly before administering medication to prevent the transfer of microorganisms to your patients.

Special handling of certain medications before administration is also important. To prevent contamination, you should avoid touching or dropping medication. For example, if you touch a topical nitrate ointment and it is accidentally absorbed through your hand, you may experience common side effects of the medication, such as headache, flushing, and hypotension. To protect your fingers from broken glass, you should place an alcohol pad around the neck of glass ampules before breaking them. Additionally, you should wear disposable gloves when administering parenteral medication to protect yourself from exposure to the patient's body fluids.

To protect patients and staff members, you must properly dispose of medications and their containers. Glass vials, ampules, needles, and syringes must be discarded in appropriate receptacles.

Any unused medications should be disposed of in the sink or toilet, and the disposal of controlled substances must be witnessed by more than one provider. Further narcotic safety includes storage in a double-locked drawer or closet. The keys to this drawer or closet (or the code to a computer-controlled dispensing system) must always be kept in the provider's possession. You should never leave these keys on top of a counter or give the computer-dispensing code to another person. If you discover a discrepancy in the inventory of controlled substances, you should report it immediately. Violations of the Controlled Substances Act are punishable by fines, imprisonment, and loss of a professional nursing license.

 To prevent sticks from contaminated needles, they should never be recapped. The keys to the double-locked drawer or closet (or the code to a computer-controlled dispensing system) must always be kept in the nurse's possession.

Remember that medications should never be left unattended or at the patient's bedside. It is your responsibility to ensure that the patient takes his or her medication as prescribed. To ensure that this is done, you should obey the six rights discussed in the following section.

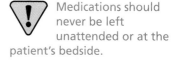 Medications should never be left unattended or at the patient's bedside.

The Right Drug

To ensure that the *right drug* is given to a patient, you must be able to recognize different medications with similar names. It is also important to verify the computerized nursing care plan or the medication administration record (MAR) with the original medication order on your patient's medical record or chart. In addition, you should check the name on the drug container against verified information and take great care to remove the correct medication from the correct drawer section of the computer-controlled dispensing system.

The Right Dose

You can ensure that the *right dose* is given by using trusted and reliable calculation procedures and double-checking your answers to make sure that they are correct. When administering medications with a narrow safety margins, such as heparin or insulin, it is important to validate the dose with another health care provider.

The Right Patient

To ensure that the *right patient* receives the medication, you must always check the patient's identification bracelet carefully with the medication order before administration. In addition, you should ask the patient to state his or her name, if possible. Keep in mind that it is inappropriate to suggest a patient's name because he or she might answer to the wrong name.

The Right Time

To ensure that the medication is administered at the *right time,* you must give it to the patient within 30 minutes of the scheduled time. Medications that need to be maintained at a consistent level in the patient's blood should given at equally distant intervals around the clock.

The Right Route

To guarantee that the right route is used, you must be sure that the drug form agrees with the medication order and that it is administered in a way that is an appropriate entry route for the medication.

Some medications require you to make special observations before administration. For example, an antihypertensive medication would require you to take a blood pressure reading before administering it to a patient. Similarly, digoxin would require you to monitor the patient's apical pulse, serum potassium, and digoxin levels before administration.

When an incorrect medication has been administered, a professional code of ethics must be followed. You should report the error to the physician and follow-up with institutional policy. Medication errors must be reported in a timely manner so that an antidote can be given to the patient as soon as possible, if necessary.

Safe medication administration also includes informing the patient about each medication being given and its use. If the patient has any unusual comments or if he or she questions the medications being given, you should always recheck the medication order to be absolutely sure of accuracy.

The Right Documentation

After a medication has been administered, you must properly document this action in the appropriate medication record. For scheduled medications, this may require only your initials. With one time or as needed prescriptions, the time of administration must be included along with your initials. It is required that you be familiar with your institution's medication documentation system.

Do You UNDERSTAND?

List the Six Rights of Medication Administration.

1. _____

2. _____

3. _____

4. _____

5. _____

6. _____

References

Cohen MR: *Medication errors: causes, prevention and risk management,* Boston, 2000, Jones and Bartlett.

DeLaune SC, Ladner PK: *Fundamentals of nursing: standards and practice,* ed 2 Albany, NY, 2002, Delmar.

Harkreader H: *Fundamentals of nursing: caring and clinical judgment,* ed 2, Philadelphia, 2004, WB Saunders.

Leahy JM, Kizilay PE: *Foundations of nursing practice: a nursing process approach,* Philadelphia, 1998, WB Saunders.

Lehne RA: *Pharmacology for nursing care,* ed 4, Philadelphia, 2004, WB Saunders.

Lindeman CA, McAthie M: *Fundamentals of contemporary nursing practice,* Philadelphia, 1999, WB Saunders.

Macklin D, Chernecky C, Infortuna H: *Math for clinical practice,* St Louis, 2005, Mosby.

Nasrawi CW, Alexander J: *Quick and easy dosage calculations,* Philadelphia, 1999, WB Saunders.

Answers: **1. Right drug, 2. Right dose, 3. Right patient, 4. Right time, 5. Right route, 6. Right documentation.**

Ogden SJ: *Calculation of drug dosages: an interactive workbook,* ed 7, St Louis, 2003, Mosby.

Potter PA, Perry AG: *Fundamentals of nursing: concepts, process, and practice,* ed 6, St Louis, 2005, Mosby.

Potter PA, Perry AG: *Basic nursing: a critical thinking approach,* ed 5, St Louis, 2005, Mosby.

NCLEX® Review

Circle the correct answer.

1. You have discovered that the pharmacy sent digoxin for a patient instead of digitoxin. To prevent compounding the error, you should:
   1 Give the medication after checking the Six Rights.
   2 Calculate a corrected dose of digoxin and administer the medication because the preparations are the same but have different strengths.
   3 Verify the correct dose with another nurse before giving the medication.
   4 Call the pharmacy and have them send up the correct medication.

2. You are transcribing the following prescription order to the medication sheet: Zantac 150 mg PO bid. What does the order mean?
   1 Administer Zantac 150 mg by mouth twice a day.
   2 Administer Zantac 150 mg by mouth every other day.
   3 Administer Zantac 75 mg twice a day, for a total of 150 mg in a 24-hour period.
   4 Administer Zantac 75 mg at 1000 hours and 2200 hours.

3. You have received the following prescription: Kefurox 1.5 g IVPB over 30 minutes. You should read this prescription order as:
   1 Administer IV Kefurox 1.5 g, with a secondary IV set over 30 minutes.
   2 Administer IV slow push Kefurox 1.5 g over 30 minutes.
   3 Administer Kefurox 1.5 g by adding it to the patient's currently hanging IV fluids.
   4 Administer IV Kefurox 1.5 g intramuscularly (IM) instead of IV.

4. Which of the following must be included in a legally valid medical prescription?
   1 Drug name and abbreviation
   2 Purpose of the medication and prescriber signature
   3 Drug name, dose, route, frequency of administration, and prescriber signature
   4 Transcribing provider's name and date written

5. To ensure accuracy when receiving a verbal or telephone order, you should:
   1 Write the prescriber's full name and indicate that the order is a verbal or telephone order.
   2 Request the same information as required in a written order.
   3 Verify the order with the licensed prescriber as it is written in the chart.
   4 Request the licensed prescriber sign the order as soon as possible.

6. While administering medications, you notice the medication ordered is digoxin 2.5 mg, and you find 0.5 mg scored tablets available. You know the safe dose range is 0.5 mg to 1.25 mg. Which of the following actions should you take?
   1 Give ½ tablet.
   2 Give 1 tablet.
   3 Give 5 tablets.
   4 Call the physician and verify the dosage.

7. The drug name that is reflective of the total content is the:
   1 Trade name
   2 Generic name
   3 Chemical name
   4 Scientific name

8. Reliable resources of drug standards and medication information include all except:
   1 *National Formulary*
   2 *British Pharmacopeia*
   3 *United States Pharmacopeia*
   4 *Physician's Desk Reference*

9. If a patient is in the bathroom when you deliver his or her medication, you should:
   1 Leave the medication on the bedside table next to the water glass.
   2 Return at a later time when the patient is able to receive the medication.
   3 Instruct the patient to take medication upon leaving the bathroom.
   4 Return the medication to the top of the medication cart until all other medications have been distributed.

10. If an incorrect medication has been given, you should:
   1 Report the error immediately upon discovery.
   2 Give the correct medication immediately.
   3 Document the correct medication as given.
   4 Report the error to the physician upon the next visit.

True or False

11. It is recommended that prescriptions be written out and that abbreviations not be used.

12. Medications either have a generic name or a trade name.

13. If a physician prescribes a medication, even if it seems unreasonable, you should administer it.

14. The first steps to administering a medication is to calculate the correct dose.

15. If the patient is asleep, it is appropriate to leave their medications on the bedside table.

NCLEX® Review Answers

1. **4** Digitalis glycosides should not be used interchangeably. Digoxin and digitoxin are digitalis glycosides but have different dosage ranges, absorption, metabolism, and half-life and should not be used interchangeably.

2. **1** PO means by mouth; *bid* means twice a day. The abbreviation for every other day is *qod*. The order for this dose would be written "Zantac 75 mg bid," and the order is for Zantac 150 mg; it does not state what time to give the medication (only that it should be given twice a day).

3. **1** *IVPB* means intravenously with a secondary IV set. The abbreviation for intravenous slow push is *IVSP*. The abbreviation for intramuscular administration is *IM*.

4. **3** Drug name, dose, route, frequency of administration, and prescriber signature must all be present for a prescription order to be legally valid. An abbreviation of the drug name is not necessary, and the purpose of the drug is not necessary for the prescription to be legally valid. The transcribing nurse's signature is also not required.

5. **3** Verifying the order with the licensed prescriber as it is written in the chart helps ensure accuracy. Writing the prescriber's full name is necessary for a valid verbal or telephone order, but it does not ensure the accuracy of the order. The request for the licensed prescriber's signature is necessary for legal validation, but it also does not ensure the accuracy of the order.

6. **4** Any time an order is questionable, the prescriber should be contacted and the order verified.

7. **2** The generic drug name is indicative of the content. Drug companies assign the trade name, which may or may not relate to drug content. The chemical name is not used to identify drugs in the hospital setting and would not necessarily relate to drug content because more than one chemical may be present in a drug. The scientific name may or may not be related to drug content.

8. **4** The *Physician's Desk Reference* is not an authoritative source of drug information. *The National Formulary, British Pharmacopeia,* and the *United States Pharmacopeia* are resources developed to ensure drug uniformity and are recognized as reliable drug standards.

9. **2** You should return and observe the Six Rights of Medication Administration. You should never leave medications unattended, you must observe the "right patient," and medications should not be returned to the unit dose container once they have been removed.

10. **1** You have a responsibility to report errors immediately, to adhere to the code of ethics, and to protect the patient so that an antidote can be administered, if necessary. Administering the correct medication after the incorrect one would put the patient in danger, and documenting the correct medication as given would violate the code of ethics and pose a potential threat to the patient. Medication errors need to be reported immediately to protect the patient and allow staff to administer any antidotes, if necessary.

11. True.

12. False. Medications have both. They have one generic name and potentially several different trade names.

13. False. If a medication order seems unreasonable, check with the pharmacy before administration.

14. False. The first step is to determine that the medication you have is the medication that has been prescribed.

15. False. Medications should never be left unattended or by the patient's bedside.

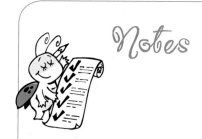

Notes

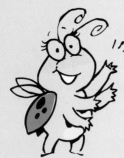

Measurement and Administration of Oral Medications

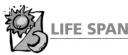

LIFE SPAN

An infant or young child will usually receive the liquid form of a drug, whereas an adult may receive the drug in capsule form. However, older adults who are unable to swallow effectively may need a crushed or liquid form of the same medication.

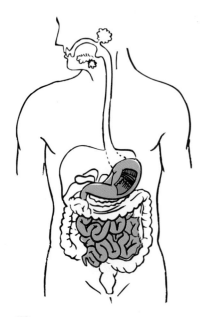

What You WILL LEARN

After reading this chapter, you will know how to do the following:

✔ Identify tablet, capsule, and liquid forms of medications.
✔ Differentiate between multiple forms of oral medications.
✔ Calculate and select appropriate medications, dosages, and methods for oral medication administration.

As a health care provider, you will administer most medications by mouth. Oral medications may be solid (i.e., tablets or capsules) or liquid preparations. They are considered the most convenient and safest form of medication. In addition, orally administered medications are generally the most economical and can be used for patients of all ages. Another advantage of oral medications is that frequently patients can self-administer them. It is important to remember that a patient's age may affect the form of oral preparation he or she receives.

Oral medications are absorbed in the gastrointestinal tract, primarily in the small intestine. Some variation in absorption may occur as a result of the presence of food in the stomach and intestines, or a variation in the pH of secretions. Because some drugs are irritating to the alimentary canal, they must be given with food; others may cause discoloration to the teeth and must be taken through a straw. Oral medications are contra-indicated when a patient is unconscious, uncooperative, unable to swallow, has gastric or intestinal suctioning, or is vomiting.

What IS a Tablet?

Tablets are powdered drug preparations that have been compressed into pills of various colors, sizes, and shapes. They are available in different forms and drug strengths. Many are scored and easily broken into halves or quarters when the amount of the drug needed is less than the amount contained in an entire tablet. Tablets may be coated (enteric coated) for various reasons—to decrease their unpleasant taste, to ease swallowing, to delay the release of medication, to protect the stomach lining (gastric mucosa), to avoid cancer-causing (carcinogenic) properties.

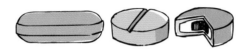

What IS a Capsule?

Capsules are hard or soft gelatin coverings that encase an oil, liquid, powder, or granular form of a specific medication. They come in a variety of colors and sizes; some have special shapes or colors that identify the company that produced them. These capsules are called *puvules*. Many capsules contain tiny spheres of medication that have been coated to ensure sustained release over a period of time. These small spheres of coated medication are called *spansules*.

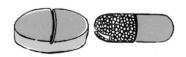

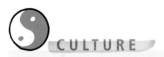
CULTURE

It is also important to remember that your Asian patients may require lower doses of psychotropic and neuroleptic medications to achieve therapeutic serum blood levels. Asians also metabolize these drugs more slowly.

TAKE HOME POINTS

Tablets coated to disguise unpleasant taste or to ease swallowing may be referred to as caplets, geltabs, gelcaps, or filmtabs.

Enteric-coated tablets must not be crushed. The enteric coating on the tablets allows them to pass through the stomach without causing irritation. They are then dissolved and absorbed in the small intestine.

You must administer capsules whole; they should never be divided, crushed, or opened. Taking this precaution helps prevent the immediate release of a large volume of the drug (which would decrease its long-term effectiveness) into the patient's system.

Medications with names containing these abbreviations should never be crushed.

Do not assume that drugs in the medication drawer or automated medication dispenser are always the correct ones.

If giving a narcotic, make sure the count is correct prior to removing the dose from the storage unit.

Always keep poured medication within your reach, and never leave it at the bedside.

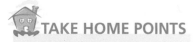

TAKE HOME POINTS

1. For patients who cannot swallow tablets or capsules, use a liquid form of the same medication when possible. For extended-release preparations, a dose adjustment may be required. Consult the pharmacist.
2. The maximum number of tablets or capsules given for one dose is usually three. Recalculate if your first calculation results in a greater number.
3. Sublingual tablets are always placed under the tongue to be absorbed. They are never swallowed.

What You NEED TO KNOW

You should be familiar with some of the common abbreviations for delayed, or extended-release tablets. Among them are the following:

CR	Controlled release
CRT	Controlled-release tablet
LA	Long acting
SR	Sustained release
TR	Time release
TD	Time delay
SA	Sustained action
XL	Extended release
XR	Extended release

To be fully prepared to give oral medications, there are a few more crucial details you must know:

- Why the patient is receiving the medications
- Usual dose range and route of medications
- Medication, dose strength, and prescribed route
- How to calculate the correct dose:

$$\frac{\text{Dose desired}}{\text{Dose on hand}} \times \text{vehicle} = \frac{\text{D}}{\text{H}} \times \text{V} = \text{Amount to give}$$

OR

- Use ratio and proportion to calculate doses:
What's available:Known = What's prescribed:Unknown
50 mg:1 tablet = 100 mg:x tablet
$50 \times x = 100$

Answer: $x = 2$ tablets

What You DO

To verify an order for accuracy:
- Compare the Medication Administration Record (MAR) or printout with the written prescription, and check the expired date of the prescription.

To obtain the correct medications:
- Use only the MAR to take the appropriate medication from the storage unit, drawer, or refrigerator.
- Compare the unit-dose package or medication label with the prescription on the MAR. If it is not identical, recheck the patient's chart. Remember, you must know generic and trade names for drugs you are giving.
- Report any discrepancy to the pharmacist.

Do You UNDERSTAND?

DIRECTIONS: **Match the following with the correct answers.**

1. _____ Caplet
2. _____ Spansule
3. _____ Enteric coated
4. _____ Capsule

a. Dissolves in the small intestine
b. Easy to swallow tablet
c. Indicates a time-release capsule
d. Drug form enclosed in a gelatin cover

DIRECTIONS: **Fill in the blanks.**

5. CR stands for _____.
6. LA stands for _____.
7. Enteric-coated tablets should never be _____.
8. Sublingual tablets must never be _____,
   but placed _____ the tongue.
9. No medication with an abbreviation indicating sustained, extended or long action, or time release should ever be _____.

What You NEED TO KNOW

Before giving any oral medication, you need to know the Six Rights of Medication Administration discussed in Chapter 4: (1) the right drug, (2) the right dose, (3) the right patient, (4) the right time, (5) the right route, and (6) right documentation.

Before administering oral medication, you should also assess for:
- Any medication allergies and hypersensitivities
- The patient's ability to swallow the solid form of the medication
- Intake and output adequacy, including npo status
- The presence of vomiting, diarrhea, bowel sounds, nasogastric or intestinal suctioning, or any circumstance affecting bowel motility or absorption of medication (e.g., recent general anesthesia, inflammatory bowel disease, history of gastrointestinal surgical resection)
- Any possibility of drug-drug or drug-food interactions

What You DO

To prepare the medication:
- Wash and dry your hands.
- If using a unit-dose system, place the unit dose as packaged into the medicine cup for transport to the patient.
- If not using a unit-dose system, pour the required number of tablets or capsules from the bottle into the lid; then transfer them to the disposable medicine cup for transport to your patient.
- Discard any dose that is dropped on the floor.
- To reduce error, recheck each medication with the MAR as you pour it.
- Keep any medication that requires a specific assessment (immediately before the medication's administration) separate from the others so that you may withhold it, if necessary.
- If a patient exhibits difficulty swallowing, crush the tablet to a fine powder with a clean pill crusher if there are no contraindications for doing so. Next, mix the powder with a small amount of soft food, such as applesauce, to ease swallowing.

- Check the MAR against the medication label for the third time to further reduce the chance of making an error.
- Keep the MAR and the prepared medication together, and avoid leaving them unattended.

To administer medication correctly:
- Identify the patient, comparing the name on the patient's identification bracelet with the name on the medication record and asking the patient his or her name. Explain the purpose of the medication in terms the patient can understand and include expected effects of the drug.
- Assist the patient to a sitting position to ease swallowing and prevent aspiration. A side-lying position may also be used if your patient is unable to sit.
- Make any required assessments, such as apical pulse rate before digitalis preparations, respiratory rate before giving narcotics, or blood pressure before giving antihypertensive drugs.
- Withhold medications if assessments fall outside prescribed parameters.
- Give the medication with sufficient water or juice.
- If the patient cannot hold the medicine cup, place it at the patient's lips and give one tablet at a time to ease swallowing and maintain cleanliness of the tablet.
- Stay with the patient until he or she has swallowed all medication (a prescription or written agency policy is required for medications to be left at the bedside).

To document each medication given:
- Record the name of medication given, dose, and time it was administered according to agency policy.
- Document any assessments made and record the results.
- Document any medication that was refused or omitted, or any complaints made by the patient concerning the medication (you should also include any actions that you took as a result of the refusal, omission, or complaint).
- Sign in the correct location.

To evaluate the effectiveness of the medication:
- Return to your patient in about 30 minutes and assess the effects of the medication you have administered.
- Document the effects you observe according to agency policy.

⚠ If the patient states that the medication you are about to give is different than what has previously been given, check the original prescription before administering the medication.

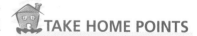

TAKE HOME POINTS

1. Verify the patient's ability to swallow and take medications by mouth.
2. Verify the prescription for accuracy.
3. Obtain the appropriate medication.
4. Prepare the medication, including the calculation of the correct dose.
5. Administer the medication.

Do You UNDERSTAND?

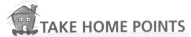

TAKE HOME POINTS

All prescriptions should be written out. For example:
PO = by mouth.
qd = every day.

DIRECTIONS: **Fill in the blanks.**

1. Inability to swallow tablets or capsules = _____.
2. Inadequate _____ _____ = less drug excretion by kidneys.
3. Before preparing a medication, _____ your hands.
4. Unit doses should be transported to the patient _____.
5. To avoid contaminating oral medications in a multi-dose bottle, pour the tablets into the _____ before pouring them into the medicine cup.
6. As medication is poured, you should only use the _____ to check it.
7. Discard any dose that is _____ on the floor.
8. Separate any medications that require an _____ assessment before administration.
9. Mix crushed tablets in _____ _____ to ease swallowing.
10. Do not leave poured medications _____.
11. Documentation is done according to agency policy, but it must always contain your _____.
12. If any medication was omitted or refused, you should document that fact and any resulting _____.
13. To evaluate the effectiveness of many medications, assess for expected outcomes after approximately _____.

DIRECTIONS: **Label the following statements *True* or *False*.**

14. _____ You do not need to check drugs in an automated dispenser for accuracy.
15. _____ You should know why a patient is receiving a certain medication.
16. _____ You should make sure the narcotic count is correct before and after removing the dose from the storage unit.

DIRECTIONS: **List three things for which the MAR is used.**

17. _____

18. _____

19. _____

DIRECTIONS: **Calculate the following:**

20. Prescribed: Zantac syrup (hydroxyzine hydrochloride) 0.05 g PO qd

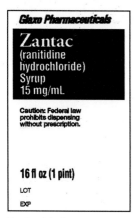

Zantac label.

Remember to change grams to milligrams by moving the decimal point three spaces to the right: 0.05 g = 0.050 g or 50 mg

Basic formula method: _____

Ratio and proportion: _____

21. Prescription: Principen (ampicillin) 500 mg PO

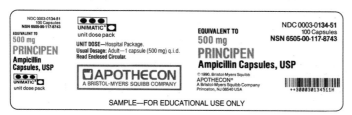

Principen label.

Basic formula method: _____

Ratio and proportion: _____

22. Prescription: digoxin (Lanoxin) 0.25 mg PO qd

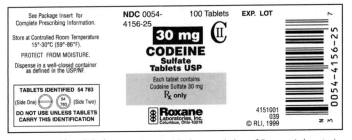

Lanoxin label.

Basic formula method: _____

Ratio and proportion: _____

23. Prescribed: Codeine sulfate gr 1 PO qoh

Codeine sulfate label. *Reproduced with the permission of Roxane Laboratories.*

Remember that gr 1 = 60 mg. Convert the grains to milligrams using ratio and proportion so that both the order and the drug as supplied are in the metric system. Then use either of the methods below to calculate the actual drug dose.

Basic formula method: _____

Ratio and proportion: _____

What IS a Liquid Medication?

Liquid medications, such as cough syrups, stool softeners, and antacids, are another type of oral medication.

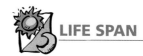

LIFE SPAN

The liquid form of a drug is often prescribed for children and older adults because it is easy to deliver orally or through a feeding tube.

What IS a Liquid Form?

A medicine that is in *liquid form* is made up of the medicine itself, called the *solute,* and the liquid added to the medicine, called the *solvent.* When the solute and solvent are combined, the result is called a *solution.* The most common solvents are water and saline solution. Liquid medication is measured using droppers or by pouring the medication into a disposable medicine cup.

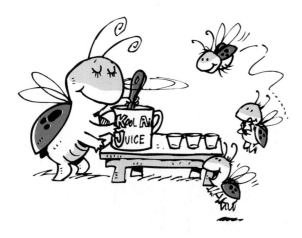

What You NEED TO KNOW

To dispense liquid medications safely, you must understand ratios and percentages (because a prescription can be written as a ratio or a percentage). For example, a ratio of 1:4 means there is 1 mL of medicine solute to 3 mL of solvent (for a total of 4 mL of solution). This is also called a ¼ strength solution. A percentage of 10% means there are 10 mL of the drug solute to 90 mL of solvent (for a total of 100 mL of solution).

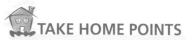

TAKE HOME POINTS

Solute + Solvent = Solution
1 mL = 1 cc
1 tsp = 5 mL
1 tbsp = 15 mL
3 tsp = 15 mL
A 1:20 solution is the same as a 5% solution

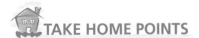

TAKE HOME POINTS

Absorption of medications is negatively affected by suction from a nasogastric tube, vomiting, or diarrhea. For patients with gastric tubes for purposes of feeding, liquid medications are preferred.

If the taste of the medication is objectionable, offer ice for 10 to 20 seconds before the medication touches the mouth and tongue. The ice makes the taste buds cold, thereby negating taste.

If medication is a narcotic, make sure the count is correct before pouring the dose.

Always have poured medication within your reach. Never leave it at the patient's bedside. It is your responsibility to make sure that the patient (not another patient) takes the medication.

TAKE HOME POINTS

Wipe the lip of the bottle with a clean paper towel before replacing the lid to keep the cap from sticking to the bottle.

Before administering a liquid medication, you should assess the patient for the following:

- Any allergies or hypersensitivities to the medication. Common liquid medications that people are often hypersensitive or allergic to include diphendydramine hydrochloride (Benadryl); cough syrups that contain codeine; docusate sodium (Colace), a stool softener; and aluminum hydroxide plus magnesium hydroxide (Maalox), an antacid.
- Patient's ability to swallow. Is he or she unconscious, confused, or suffering from a neuromuscular disease, stomatitis, or esophageal stricture?
- Presence of vomiting or diarrhea.
- Reduced motility or diminished bowel sounds (due to general anesthesia, bowel inflammation, or surgical gastrointestinal resection).
- Nothing by mouth (npo) status.
- Presence of a nasogastric tube to suction.
- Patient's ability to understand the purpose of the medication being administered.
- Expiration dates of the medications being given.

When administering liquid medications, also remember the following:

- Before giving any medication, always read the prescription and medication label, ask the patient his or her name, and check the patient's arm band to verify the name given.
- Check to see whether the medication has an objectionable taste by asking your patient if he or she has received the medication before, or try a small amount on the patient's tongue and watch for a negative reaction.
- If the volume of medication required is less than 10 mL, obtain a 10 mL syringe (without a needle) and use it as the measurement device.

Nursing care regarding planning and evaluation is necessary for comprehensive patient care.

- Give the patient ice orally 10 to 20 seconds before dispensing bad-tasting oral medications to help reduce a negative reaction.
- Sign out for all medications, including narcotics.
- Evaluate the effectiveness of medications within 30 minutes.

Age-Specific Considerations

When administering liquid medications to the older adult, you should consider physiologic changes that can influence the administration and effectiveness of oral medications. These changes include decreased vision and impaired memory that influence self-administration of medications, decreased renal function (slowing elimination and increasing drug concentration in bloodstream over long periods), and slower gastrointestinal absorption (influencing the effectiveness of medications).

When administering liquid medications to infants and children, it is acceptable to retrieve and readminister medication when an infant pushes a medicine spoon away. If possible, it may be necessary to dilute a liquid medication using a small amount of water or a nonessential food item, such as jelly, honey, or fruit puree. Use of essential food items, such as cereal or orange juice, to dilute medications can cause the child to develop an aversion to these foods; it is not recommended.

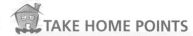

TAKE HOME POINTS

1. Do NOT describe medicine as food or as a treat; describe it as a medicine.
2. To prevent nausea, offer less than 10 cc of a carbonated beverage before and after administering oral medication.
3. To prevent an unpleasant taste, offer licks of a popsicle before and after administering oral medication.

What You DO

Nursing knowledge and interventions are based on years of practice and research. Consider the following nursing interventions for liquid medications:

- Feeding tubes (nasogastric, J, G-tubes only) should be checked for proper position and then irrigated with 50 to 150 mL of room-temperature water before giving medication. Do this again after administering the medication through the tube.
- Crushed tablets and soft-gel capsules should be dissolved in at least 60 mL of warm water to ensure a completely dissolved solution.
- When in doubt about crushing medications, consult a pharmacist (see table on the following page).
- To pour medication, hold the medication cup at eye level and fill to the correct level using the bottom of the meniscus (the crescent-shaped portion at the top of the liquid).

Some medications come in popsicle form (e.g., chlorpheniramine maleate [Chlor-Trimeton]). The child must finish the entire popsicle to get the correct dose.

When using a syringe to dispense liquid medication, place the syringe to the side of the tongue to prevent choking and aspiration.

If children are taking sweetened medication for more than 10 days, begin oral hygiene following administration to prevent cavities.

Avoid giving syrups or medications with a pH that is less than 4 because this acidity creates gastrointestinal distress. Check the drug package insert or call a pharmacist for specific pH information.

Do not give patients whole, undissolved, or medications that should not be crushed through a gastric tube.

TAKE HOME POINTS

1. To enhance ingestion and prevent aspiration, have your patient sit up. If this is not possible, a side-lying position will also work.
2. Obtain bottled medication and note expiration date, patient name, dose, and route.
3. Pour medication away from the label to prevent damaging written information.
4. If the volume of medication is less than 10 cc, use a syringe (without needle) to draw the medication.

Common Medications That Should Not Be Crushed

TRADE NAME	GENERIC NAME
Cardizem	diltiazem hydrochloride
Depakote	divalproex sodium valproic acid
EES	erythromycin ethylsuccinate
E-mycin	erythromycin base
Erythromycin	erythromycin estolate
Feosol	ferrous sulfate
Glucotrol XL	glipizide
Klor-con	potassium chloride
K-tab	potassium chloride
MS Contin	morphine sulfate
Phazyme	simethicone
Prilosec	omeprazole
Prozac	fluoxetine hydrochloride
Slow-K	potassium chloride
Theobid	theophylline
Theo-Dur	theophylline

Do You UNDERSTAND?

DIRECTIONS: **Fill in the blanks.**

1. Solute + _____ = solution
2. 3 tsp = _____ mL
3. 5 mL = _____ cc
4. 2 tbsp = _____ mL
5. A one-half strength solution is 50% solvent plus _____ solute.
6. A one-half strength solution means adding 75 cc of water to _____ _____ cc of medication.

DIRECTIONS: **List two types of medications you should not crush.**

7. _____

8. _____

9. Color in the syringe amount for 1 teaspoon of medication.

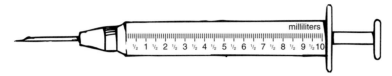

10. Circle the picture that has the correct amount of 30 cc of medication.

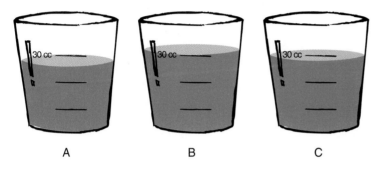

A   B   C

11. Which food item is most appropriate for medication mixture?
    a. Apple juice
    b. Jelly
    c. Cereal

References

Bartels D: Clinical practice. Adherence to oral therapy for type 2 diabetes: opportunities for enhancing glycemic control, *J Am Acad Nurse Pract* 16(1):8-16, 2004.

Birner A: Pharmacology of oral chemotherapy agents, *Clin J Oncol Nurs* 7(6): Oral chemotherapy: considerations for oncology nursing practice, 11-9, 37-9, 2003.

Cabaleiro J: Flavoring meds for children and adults: so it goes down easy! *Home Health Nurs* 21(5):295-8, 2003.

Gray DC: *Calculate with confidence,* ed 2, St Louis, 1998, Mosby.

Kee JL, Hayes ER: *Pharmacology: a nursing process approach,* ed 2, Philadelphia, 1997, WB Saunders.

Kozier B et al: *Fundamentals of nursing: concepts, process, and practice,* ed 5, Menlo Park, Calif, 1998, Addison-Wesley.

Ogden S: *Calculation of drug dosages: an interactive workbook,* ed 6, St Louis, 1999, Mosby.

Answer: 9. 1 tsp = 5 mL; 10. b; 11. b.

Notes

NCLEX® Review

Circle the correct answer.

1. Colace (docusate sodium) is a medicine that is added to a liquid to form an oral solution. Colace, the additive medicine, is known as the:
   1 Solvent
   2 Solute
   3 Solution
   4 Irrigant

2. Mrs. Koo is to receive a total of 8 teaspoons of cough syrup, in equally divided doses, every 6 hours for 24 hours. You are to give her the first dose at 0600 hours. How many milliliters of cough medicine would you pour for her first dose?
   1 5
   2 10
   3 15
   4 30

3. Mr. Rodriguez is unconscious, has a nasogastric tube, and has been prescribed enteric-coated aspirin (325 mg) to be given now. Your best intervention is to:
   1 Crush the medication and give it to Mr. Rodriguez via his nasogastric tube.
   2 Give the medication rectally since Mr. Rodriguez is unconscious.
   3 Call the pharmacist for liquid aspirin so you can give it by mouth via a syringe.
   4 Call the physician who prescribed the medication for a more appropriate prescription.

4. Mr. MacGuinness is 84 years old and has just been prescribed six different medications by two different physicians. Which of Mr. MacGuinness' organs should you assess in relation to the body's elimination of the medications prescribed?
   1 Bone marrow
   2 Kidneys

   3 Brain
   4 Lungs

5. Which one of the following patients would probably have decreased gastrointestinal motility and therefore not effectively absorb a liquid medication. A patient who:
   1 Just had a gastrointestinal resection 8 hours earlier
   2 Is without teeth
   3 Is sitting upright
   4 Is preparing for a chest x-ray film

6. The physician prescribes Cardizem (diltiazem HCL) 60 mg for Mr. Kitchens. You have 30 mg tablets in stock. How many tablets should he receive?
   1 0.5 tablet
   2 1 tablet
   3 1.5 tablets
   4 2 tablets

7. The physician prescribes Augmentin 0.875 g PO q12h for Mrs. Yang. You have Augmentin 875 mg in stock. How many tablets should you give Mrs. Yang?
   1 0.5 tablet
   2 1 tablet
   3 2 tablets
   4 3 tablets

8. The physician prescribes codeine gr ¾ for Mr. Walenski q4h prn for pain. You have 30 mg tablets in stock. How many tablets should you give Mr. Walenski?
   1 ¼ tablet
   2 ¾ tablet
   3 1½ tablets
   4 2 tablets

9. The physician prescribes Lopid (gemfibrozil) 600 mg for Mr. Smith. You have received a unit dose labeled Lopid 0.6 g from the pharmacy. What action should you take?
   1 Give the unit dose as sent from the pharmacy.
   2 Withhold the dose until the physician is consulted.
   3 Call the pharmacy to report a mistake in the dose.
   4 Return the medication to the pharmacy.

10. The pharmacy sends up a certain medication in capsule form. You calculate that the patient is to receive one half of a capsule. What action should you take before administering the medication?
    1 Break the capsule open and administer one half of the contents.
    2 Consult the pharmacist for a liquid form of the drug.
    3 Verify that the dosage calculation was correct.
    4 Mix the contents of the capsule in 30 cc of water and administer 15 cc to the patient.

11. True or False? It is good nursing practice if you crush time released (TR) medication tablets so the elderly patient can take them.

12. Short answer: Your patient states they are allergic to Loracarbef (Lorabid) an antibiotic used to treat urinary tract infections and a medication of the carbacephem class of antibiotics. This patient has a urinary tract infection and is prescribed the antibiotic levofloxacin (Levaquin), a medication of the fluoroquinolone class of antibiotics. Should you give the Levaquin to your patient?

13. True or False? You have poured 15 mL of a liquid medication and the patient refuses to take it. You should chart the refusal but save the medication until the end of your shift in case the patient decides to change his/her mind and take the medication.

14. True or False? You should pour liquid medication away from the label.

15. Fill in the blank: Prevent giving syrups or medication with a pH less than _____ because this acidity creates gastrointestinal distress.

NCLEX® Review Answers

1. **2** Solute is the additive. Solvent is the liquid added to the medicine. Solution is the solvent plus the solute. Irrigant is usually used to wash wounds or flush tubes.

2. **2** 8 tsp/24 hr = 2 tsp/6 hr 1tsp = 5 mL so 2 tsp = 10 ml.

3. **4** You should not crush enteric-coated medications, and enteric-coated tablets are not appropriate for the rectal route. In addition, if the patient is unconscious; you should not give him anything by mouth.

4. **2** The kidneys are the organs of elimination. Bone marrow is where red blood cells, white blood cells, and platelets are made. The brain is the organ of thinking and reasoning. The lungs are responsible for breathing.

5. **1** Surgery decreases gastrointestinal motility because anesthesia is used. Teeth do not influence gastrointestinal motility. Sitting upright increases digestion. Preparing for a chest x-ray requires no change in eating habits and does not influence gastrointestinal motility.

6. **4** 60 mg:1 = 30 mg:x, so 60 ÷ 30 = 2.

7. **2** 0.875 g = 875 mg, because 1000 mg = 1 g. Therefore, 1 tablet.

8. **3** 1 gr = 60 mg, so 0.75 gr:x mg (or ¾:x mg) = 1 gr: 60 mg and x = 45 mg. With 30-mg tablets, you will need 1½ tablets to give the patient 45 mg.

9. **1** 1000 mg = 1 g, so 600 mg = 0.6 g. The unit dose is correct. There is no mistake; these doses are the same, and there's no need to return the medication to the pharmacy.

10. **3** Verifying the dose would be your first action (capsules are usually not to be opened). Consulting the pharmacist for a liquid form would be appropriate, but it would not be your first action. In addition, you always validate doses before mixing contents (if appropriate).

11. False. Crushing voids the time-released property of the tablet.

12. Yes. These two antibiotics may sound somewhat alike but they are a different class of antibiotics; hence the history of allergies does not apply to the prescribed antibiotic.

13. False. Waste the medication.

14. True. This prevents damaging the label.

15. 4.

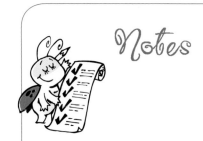

Notes

6 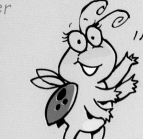 Intramuscular Drugs

What You WILL LEARN

After reading this chapter, you will know how to do the following:
- ✔ Define intramuscular injection.
- ✔ Use safety measures in determining dosages for intramuscular medications.
- ✔ Calculate volumes of prescribed dosages for intramuscular injections.

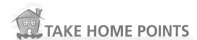

TAKE HOME POINTS

Six Rights of Medication Administration
1. The right drug
2. The right dose
3. The right patient
4. The right time
5. The right route
6. Right documentation

Intramuscular (IM) injections, are used to administer analgesics, antibiotics, antihistamines, vaccines, steroidal antiinflammatory medications, and other medications. When a patient requires increased medication absorption and response that cannot be obtained through the use of oral medications, IM injections may be used. Patients who are unable to swallow, who are allowed nothing by mouth (NPO), or who have a gastrointestinal condition that hinders their absorption of medications may also be given IM injections. Because this form of medication administration bypasses the gastrointestinal tract, IM injections may also be referred to as *parenteral injections.*

Giving IM injections safely requires knowledge and skill. This chapter covers the essentials of administering medications safely by this route.

What IS a Safety Measure?

Proper *safety measures* ensure that no one is injured by an accidental needle stick. By following the Six Rights of Medication Administration, drawing up medications yourself, administering them correctly, and disposing of used needles and syringes appropriately, you will ensure the safety of your patients, yourself, and others.

What You NEED TO KNOW

Accidental needle sticks and other needle-related injuries can occur in health care settings. Needle sticks commonly occur when health care providers recap needles or come in contact with needles left at the patient's bedside. Safety syringe systems that protect the needle after medication is drawn up and after patient usage are required. Needle protection guidelines require that needles are never recapped and always disposed of in a sharps containers.

What You DO

When using needles, special care must be taken. Understanding how to correctly use the institution's needleless system is very important. Always dispose of syringes in a sharps container immediately after use.

You must dispose of all used needles and syringes in sharps containers; they must never be left at the patient's bedside or placed in a wastebasket, your pocket, or other "convenient" spot.

Do You UNDERSTAND?

DIRECTIONS: Circle the items that help prevent the transmission of bloodborne disease when using needles.

Sharps boxes	Safety guards on needles
Needleless devices	Wastebaskets
Provider's pockets	Patient's bedcovers

Answers: **1. Sharps boxes, needleless devices, safety guards on needles.**

TAKE HOME POINTS

1. Do not try to force a needle into a full sharps box (this is one of the most common ways to get a needle stick).
2. Do not administer a medication that has been drawn up by another provider.

What IS an Intramuscular Injection?

Intramuscular (IM) *injections* are given into muscle under the subcutaneous tissue. A medication is introduced using a syringe and a needle long enough to go through the dermis and subcutaneous tissue and into the body of the muscle.

What You NEED TO KNOW

The size, also known as the *gauge* (circumference of the needle), of catheter and the length of the needle selected for an IM injection depend on three things: (1) the type and viscosity (thickness) of medication injected, (2) the weight of the person being injected, and (3) the site chosen for the injection. You must choose a needle with a gauge large enough to allow the medication to be injected easily and long enough to reach the targeted muscle.

The usual gauge size for IM injections ranges from 19 to 23 gauge, depending on the viscosity of the medication. The greater the viscosity, the larger the gauge needs to be (the smaller the gauge number). For IM injections given to adults, a needle length of 1, $1\frac{1}{2}$, or 2 inches is usually required, depending on the amount of subcutaneous tissue.

It is important to remember that women generally have more subcutaneous tissue than men. For women weighing under 132 pounds, a $\frac{5}{8}$-inch length needle is generally adequate to penetrate the deltoid muscle. However, for women between 132 and 198 lb, a 1-inch length needle is usually required. For women weighing more than 198 lb, a $1\frac{1}{2}$-inch length needle may be necessary. For men weighing between 130 and 259 lb, a 1-inch length needle is usually adequate for IM injections into the deltoid muscle.

Medications for injection come as a liquid or powder and are packaged in several forms, including:

- Small glass containers (e.g., ampules) with narrow necks
- Prefilled cartridges
- Single-dose vials (e.g., glass containers with rubber stoppers at the top)
- Multiple-dose vials

If a vial contains a powder that must be reconstituted, directions for the volume and type of diluent are usually printed on the vial's label or on the package insert for the medication (see Chapter 7).

What You DO

To draw up a medication from an ampule:
- Hold the ampule upright and tap it gently with a finger until all the liquid is below the ampule neck. Another method to clear the top of the ampule is to hold the neck firmly between the thumb and middle finger while placing the end of the index finger on the bottom of the ampule.
- Lift your arm and swing the ampule in a downward motion to force the liquid into the bottom of the ampule.
- Once the ampule neck is clear, clean the neck of the ampule with an alcohol swab.
- Using the same swab or a 2 × 2 gauze pad, snap the top off the ampule in a direction that is away from your face to prevent the possibility of glass particles flying into your eyes.
- Without touching the ampule rim, aspirate the ordered volume of the medication into the syringe using a filter needle to prevent aspiration of glass particles into the syringe.
- Invert the syringe, clear the air bubbles by tapping on the syringe until they float to the top, then expel them.

Discard filter needle in sharps container and apply an appropriate needle for administration.

To draw up a medication from a vial:
- Swab the stopper with alcohol and allow it to dry.
- Inject air equal to the volume of the prescribed dose into the vial.
- Invert the vial and syringe as a single unit, and make sure the tip of the needle is below the fluid level.
- Allow the syringe to fill to the prescribed dose.
- Gently tap the syringe barrel to allow air bubbles to float to the top, then expel them.

Recent research indicates that when a disposable plastic syringe is used, it is not necessary to draw up a small air bubble to prevent tracking of medication through subcutaneous tissue when the needle is withdrawn because the syringe is manufactured to eliminate the need for an air bubble.

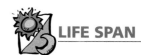

LIFE SPAN

A well-developed adult can tolerate up to 3 mL of medication given into a large muscle without undue discomfort. Older children, very slender adults, and older adults can tolerate up to 2 mL. No more than 1 mL should be given IM to older infants and toddlers.

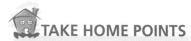

TAKE HOME POINTS

When adding a diluent to a multiple-dose vial, write the date, time, and your initials on the vial's label.

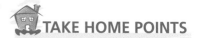

TAKE HOME POINTS

1. Always snap the top of a vial away from your face to prevent the possibility of glass particles flying into your eyes.
2. Use a filter needle to draw up medication from a vial to prevent aspiration of glass particles into the syringe.

Do You UNDERSTAND?

DIRECTIONS: **List the types of medications that may be given IM in the flower petals.**

1. Choose from the following: analgesics, antihistamines, antibiotics, chemotherapeutic medications, immunizations, steroidal antiinflammatory medications, purified protein derivative (PPD).

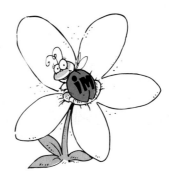

DIRECTIONS: **Match the descriptions in Column A with the appropriate needle in Column B.**

Column A	Column B
2. _____ Thin man	a. 1½-inch needle
3. _____ Thick medication	b. 20-gauge needle
4. _____ Overweight woman	c. 1-inch needle
5. _____ Watery medication	d. 23-gauge needle

DIRECTIONS: **Label the following statements *True* or *False*.**

6. _____ Ampules are glass, single-dose containers with narrow necks.

7. _____ You should snap off ampule tops toward the face to prevent finger nicks.

8. _____ You should inject air into ampules before withdrawing the desired dose of a medication.

9. _____ To clear air from the syringe, you should tap it to allow bubbles to float to the top, then expel them.

10. _____ You should inject air into a vial before withdrawing the desired dose of a medication.

What You NEED TO KNOW

Premixed medication solutions are stored in vials, ampules, and prefilled cartridges. The label on the container gives the medication dose in the container by strength and its equivalent volume (mL). For example, the following label shows Amikin 500 mg/2 mL.

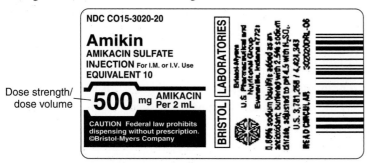

Amikin label.

If a health care practitioner prescribes Amikin 250 mg IM, you can use either the formula method or ratio-proportion method (see Chapter 5) to calculate the prescribed dose. Example:

Basic formula: $\dfrac{D}{H} \times V = \dfrac{250\ mg}{500\ mg} \times 2\ mL = \dfrac{500}{500} = 1\ mL$

Ratio-proportion method:

$$\dfrac{500\ mg}{2\ mL} = \dfrac{250\ mg}{x\ mL} \qquad 500x = 250 \times 2$$

$$x = \dfrac{500}{500}$$

$$x = 1\ mL$$

Injectable medications, although stored in different containers, may sometimes be mixed in the same syringe when compatible. To determine compatibility, consult a medication reference or a pharmacist. Compatibility tables are also available from medication manufacturers, and they may be displayed in the medication preparation area or health care practitioner's office.

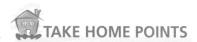

TAKE HOME POINTS

When in doubt about medication compatibility, DO NOT mix medications in the same syringe.

What You DO

To mix medications from two vials in the same syringe:

- Clean the stopper of both vials and inject air (in the volume of the solution to be withdrawn) into the first vial. Do not allow the needle to touch the solution in the vial.
- Inject air (in the volume of the solution to be withdrawn) into the second vial. Invert it and withdraw the desired volume of solution.
- If you are not using the entire volume in the first vial, change the needle to prevent contaminating the remainder of the solution (syringes with permanently attached needles will make this impossible).
- Invert the first vial and withdraw the desired volume of solution.

To mix two medications in a syringe from a vial and an ampule:

- Clean the stopper and inject air into the vial in the volume of the solution to be withdrawn.
- Withdraw the desired volume of the solution from the vial.
- Withdraw the desired volume of solution from the ampule. If available, a filter needle should be used. However, you must change the needle before injecting the patient.

To mix two medications when one is a prefilled cartridge and the other is in a vial:

- Check the volume of solution necessary to administer the dose of the medication in the prefilled cartridge. Expel any excess solution.
- Draw air into the cartridge in the volume of the solution to be withdrawn from the vial.
- Clean the stopper, invert the vial, and inject the air.
- Carefully withdraw only the desired volume of solution from the vial, making sure that the needle bevel remains beneath the fluid.

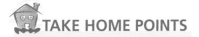

TAKE HOME POINTS

After withdrawing medication from a vial, change the needle before injecting the patient to ensure needle sharpness.

Do You UNDERSTAND?

DIRECTIONS: Answer the following for IM injections.

1. Prescribed: Rocephin 50 mg intramuscular (IM). Working with the label below, determine how many milliliters of Rocephin you should administer to your patient.

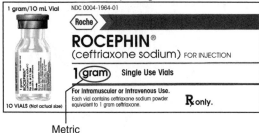

1 gram/10 mL Vial   NDC 0004-1964-01

(Roche)

ROCEPHIN®
(ceftriaxone sodium) FOR INJECTION

1 gram   Single Use Vials

For Intramuscular or Intravenous Use.
Each vial contains ceftriaxone sodium powder
equivalent to 1 gram ceftriaxone.   **R** only.

10 VIALS (Not actual size)

Metric

Rocephin label.

2. Prescribed: Demerol 50 mg and Vistaril 25 mg IM. These two medications are compatible. Both medications are in single dose vials. Give directions to mix the medications in the cartridge.

_____

_____

_____

_____

_____

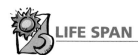

LIFE SPAN

For adults and children over the age of 7 months, you should choose the ventrogluteal site (i.e., gluteus medius, or hip) because no injuries are associated with this site, and it is easy to find.

What You NEED TO KNOW

For an IM injection, choose a site that is free of tenderness, bloody discoloration under the skin (i.e., ecchymosis), any hardened lesions, lymph edema, infection, or necrosis. Use a site that is not close to major nerves and blood vessels.

The most common sites are ventrogluteal and dorsogluteal. Other sites that may be used for IM injections are the vastus lateralis (anterior lateral thigh), the deltoid (upper arm), and the rectus femoris (anterior thigh). Because it is so accessible, the rectus femoris is most often used for self-injections (see Table 6-1, p. 104).

Answers: 0.5 mL; 2. **Clean the stopper of both vials and inject air** (in the volume of the solution to be withdrawn) into the first vial. Do not allow the needle to touch the solution in the vial. Inject air (in the volume of the solution to be withdrawn) into the second vial. Invert it and withdraw the desired volume of solution. Invert the first vial and withdraw the desired volume of solution.

! The dorsogluteal (upper, outer quadrant of the buttock) is a traditional site for IM injections. However, it has been associated with injuries to the sciatic nerve and may be difficult to find if the patient has sagging, flabby tissue in the area. Therefore you should consider the ventrogluteal site first.

What You DO

To locate the ventrogluteal site:

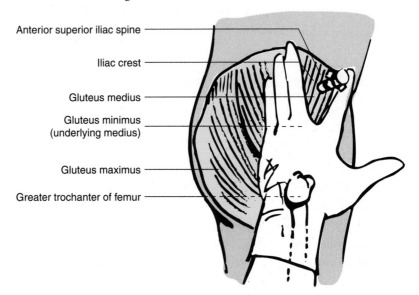

Anterior superior iliac spine

Iliac crest

Gluteus medius

Gluteus minimus
(underlying medius)

Gluteus maximus

Greater trochanter of femur

- Place the heel of your hand over the greater trochanter of the hip with your wrist perpendicular to the femur. Your right hand is used for the left hip, and your left hand is used for the right hip.
- Point your thumb toward the patient's groin, and place your index finger at the anterior superior iliac spine.
- Extend your middle finger back along the iliac crest toward the buttock until the index finger, the middle finger, and the iliac crest form a v-shaped triangle. The injection site is the center of the triangle.

The dorsogluteal site is the upper, outer quadrant of the buttock, but it may be difficult to locate because of obscured landmarks. In view of the disadvantages related to using this site for IM injections, this site is not recommend for use.

To locate the vastus lateralis site:

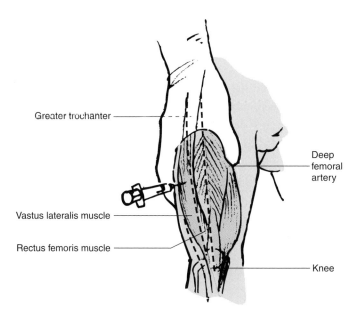

- Place one hand on the anterior lateral (outside front) of the leg above the knee and the other at the greater trochanter of the femur. The space between the hands (the middle third of the muscle) is the appropriate site of injection. When using this site for very slender adults or young children, grasp the body of the muscle to be sure the medication penetrates it.

To locate the deltoid site:

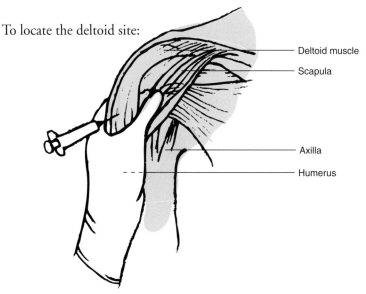

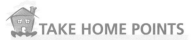

TAKE HOME POINTS

Completely expose the deltoid if it is used. Have the patient remove his or her shirt, if necessary. Inject into the center of the muscle.

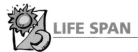

LIFE SPAN

- For infants under 7 months, the vastus lateralis site is preferred because that muscle is more developed than other potential sites.
- Do not lie to children about what will happen. Explain the injection as a little pinch that will be over in a few seconds.
- Do not prepare an injection or clear air from a syringe in front of a patient of any age. This practice causes needless anxiety and dread.
- For older adults or for adults who weigh above average and have flabby, sagging buttocks, do not use the dorsogluteal site.
- Because the deltoid muscle is not well developed in children, avoid it as an injection site.
- Only use the deltoid site in adults when small volumes of a medication are necessary.

- Find the lower edge of the acromion process at the midpoint of the lateral aspect of the upper arm.
- Measure an area below the achromion process that is three fingers wide, and outline the deltoid muscle with your thumb and fingers to its insertion site. The middle of the resulting triangle is the injection site. In adults, the deltoid site should only be used if it is well developed. It is suitable for injections of 1 cc or less.

To give a standard IM injection:
- Explain the procedure to the patient. Include exactly what will be done, where the injection will be given, how the injection will feel, and why the injection is necessary. Include the name and purpose of the medication being given, and ask again about any medication allergies.
- Locate the desired IM injection site using anatomic landmarks, and clean it with an antiseptic swab.
- Spread the skin and insert the needle quickly into the muscle at a 90-degree angle to reduce discomfort.
- Aspirate (i.e., pull back on) the plunger to be sure the needle is not lodged in a blood vessel. Use your palm to stabilize the needle while aspirating with the nondominant hand to prevent movement of the needle while in the patient.
- If blood appears, withdraw the needle, discard the medication, and prepare a new injection.
- If no blood appears, inject the medication slowly.
- Withdraw the needle smoothly and quickly while placing an antiseptic swab or dry gauze pad over the site.
- Gently massage the site to enhance absorption of the medication. Avoid vigorous massage because it may cause tissue damage.
- Assess the site for bleeding and apply pressure as necessary.
- Assist the patient to a comfortable position, and dispose of the used needle and syringe in an approved container.
- Observe the patient for adverse effects immediately following the injection and for up to 30 minutes afterward. Remember that medication reactions may occur soon after IM injection because the medication is usually absorbed rapidly.

To give a Z-track IM injection:
The Z-track method is used to minimize irritation and staining at an IM injection site. It seals the medication in the muscle tissue and prevents

back flow into subcutaneous tissue. This method is recommended for all IM injections, but it is particularly useful when administering medications that irritate or stain the skin.

- Draw up the medication from a vial or ampule using sterile technique.
- Change the needle to be sure that no medication remains on the outside of the needle shaft.
- Select a site with a well-developed muscle.
- Prepare the site with antiseptic, and pull the overlying skin and subcutaneous tissue about 1 to 1½ inches to the side.
- Hold the skin to the side with your nondominant hand, and insert the needle deep into the muscle.
- Aspirate using the fingers of the hand holding the syringe.
- If there is no blood return upon aspiration, inject the medication slowly to allow even dispersion of the medication into the muscle tissue. If blood appears in the syringe, withdraw the needle, discard the medication, and start over.
- Withdraw the needle and release the skin as it is withdrawn. The skin will slide over and form a zigzag path, or Z-track, that covers the site of the needle stick in the muscle. This Z-track ensures that the medication cannot escape into the subcutaneous tissue or to the skin surface.

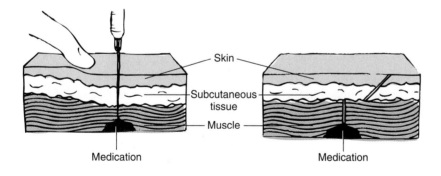

- To prevent medication seepage into the subcutaneous tissue, do not massage the injection site.

When documenting an IM injection, include the date and time given, the medication and dose administered, the reason for administration, the specific site of injection, and the patient's reaction. If pain medication was administered, don't forget to document its effectiveness.

Do You UNDERSTAND?

DIRECTIONS: **Circle indications for rejecting a site for an IM injection.**

1. Close to blood vessels   Necrotic area

   Far from major nerves   Hard lump

   Free of tenderness   Freckled skin

DIRECTIONS: **Circle the best site for an IM injection for an unconscious adult who is receiving 1½ mL of an antibiotic.**

2. Rectus femoris   Dorsogluteal

   Ventrogluteal   Deltoid

DIRECTIONS: **Label the following statements *True* or *False*.**

3. _____   To locate the patient's right ventrogluteal IM site, use your left hand to find the landmarks.

4. _____   The middle third of the inside front of the leg is the site of the vastus lateralis IM injection site.

5. _____   The deltoid IM site is located midway between the shoulder and the elbow on the lateral aspect of the arm.

DIRECTIONS: **Fill in the blanks.**

6. The Z-track method prevents _____
   of irritating or staining medications into subcutaneous tissues.

7. Skin should be pulled aside about _____ inches
   when using the Z-track method.

8. After injecting the medication, withdraw the needle and _____
   _____ the skin to make a zigzag path.

DIRECTIONS: **Fill in the blanks.**

9. When giving an IM injection, insert the needle quickly to _____

_____.

10. If blood appears upon aspiration, _____,

_____, and _____.

11. After withdrawing the needle, gentle massage may be applied to

_____.

12. Vigorous massage of the injection site after IM injection may

_____.

13. Observe the patient for medication reactions up to 30 minutes

after an IM injection has been given because _____

_____.

Table 6-1 Common Intramuscular Injection Sites

Muscle	Location	Patient Position	Advantages	Disadvantages
Ventrogluteal	Hip, just below iliac crest	Back, side, or abdomen with hip and knee flexed	Used for all patients Free of large blood vessels and nerves Less fatty tissue Not painful to lie on injection site Z-track method may be used Easily identified	Needle may touch bone
Dorsogluteal	Upper, outer quadrant of buttock	On side, with hip and knee flexed or prone with toes pointed inward	Z-track method may be used	Can be used with adults only Close to sciatic nerve Fatty tissue may obscure site Longer needle is required Injuries have been reported
Vastus lateralis	Outer, middle third of thigh	Supine or sitting	Good site for adults, children, and infants Does not lie over a joint No large nerves or blood vessels in area Well developed in infants	Leg muscles must be relaxed
Rectus femoris	Middle of top of thigh	Supine or sitting	Well developed Can be used in adults, children, and infants Fairly easy to locate	Causes pain; to be used only if other sites cannot be used
Deltoid	Lateral aspect of upper arm	Supine or sitting		It is small; cannot inject more than 1 mL May not be used in infants Arm must be relaxed

References

Curren AM, Munday LD: *Math for meds: dosages and solutions,* ed 8, San Diego, 2004, WI Publications.

Harkreader H: *Fundamentals of nursing: caring and clinical judgment,* Philadelphia, 2000, WB Saunders.

Kee JL, Hayes ER: *Pharmacology: a nursing process approach,* ed 4, Philadelphia, 2004, WB Saunders.

Lindman CA, McAthie M: *Fundamentals of contemporary nursing practice,* Philadelphia, 1999, WB Saunders.

Macklin D, Chernecky C, Infortuna H: *Math for clinical practice,* St Louis, 2005, Mosby.

Poland GA et al: Determination of deltoid fat pad thickness: implications for needle length in adult immunization, *JAMA* 277:1709, 1997.

Potter PA, Perry AG: *Basic nursing: a critical thinking approach,* ed 6, St Louis, 2005, Mosby.

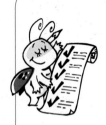

Notes

NCLEX® Review

Circle the correct answer.

1. You have been asked to administer gentamicin 60 mg IM and have a vial of gentamicin labeled 80 mg/2 mL. How many milliliters should you give the patient?
   1 0.5 mL
   2 1 mL
   3 1.25 mL
   4 1.5 mL

2. When mixing two medications in the same syringe from a vial and an ampule, you should:
   1 Remove solution from the vial first.
   2 Remove solution from the ampule first.
   3 Inject air into the ampule before removing the solution.
   4 Avoid mixing two medications in the same syringe.

3. You must give atropine sulfate 0.2 mg IM. Atropine sulfate is available in a 20-mL vial containing 0.4 mg/mL. How many milliliters should you administer to the patient?
   1 2 mL
   2 0.5 mL
   3 0.2 mL
   4 1 mL

4. The best IM site for most adults is the:
   1 Deltoid
   2 Ventrogluteal
   3 Dorsogluteal
   4 Vastus lateralis

5. The Z-track method of giving IM injections:
   1 Prevents seepage of medications into the subcutaneous (SubQ) tissue
   2 Cannot be used in the ventrogluteal site

3 Does not require you to aspirate for blood
   4 Eliminates injection discomfort for the patient

6. Recapping of used needles:
   1 Is never done under any circumstances
   2 Is no longer an option, since needleless devices are used
   3 Is only done in an emergency situation if you cannot get to a sharps box
   4 Can be done at your convenience

7. The best technique to minimize pain during injections is to:
   1 Insert the needle steadily, inject the medication quickly, and withdraw slowly.
   2 Insert the needle quickly, inject the medication slowly, and withdraw quickly.
   3 Insert the needle quickly, inject the medication quickly, and withdraw slowly.
   4 Insert the needle quickly, inject the medication quickly, and massage the site vigorously.

8. A patient about to receive a ventrogluteal injection may be placed in which of the following positions to facilitate the injection?
   1 On the back
   2 On the side
   3 On the abdomen
   4 All of the above

9. You must give a patient 500,000 Units of procaine penicillin, a very viscous medication. Which is the best gauge needle for this injection?
   1 18 gauge
   2 21 gauge
   3 22 gauge
   4 28 gauge

10. You have calculated that Mr. Amacker, a well-developed 40-year-old man, is to receive ½ mL of flu vaccine IM. Based on the volume to be given and thin viscosity of the solution, the best site to give this vaccine is the:
    1 Vastus lateralis
    2 Deltoid
    3 Dorsogluteal
    4 Ventrogluteal

Fill in the Blanks

11. Select the gauge of the catheter based on the _____ _____ of the medicine.

12. Select the length of the catheter based on _____ _____ and _____.

13. Because IM injections bypass the gastrointestinal tract they are also referred to as _____ _____.

True or False

14. It is best to rub the injection site vigorously after an IM injection to minimize pain and disperse the medication evenly in the muscle.

15. With Z track injections you must change the needle after drawing up the medication before administration.

NCLEX® Review Answers

1. **4** $\frac{80}{2} = \frac{60}{x}$, $80x = 120$, $x = \frac{120}{180}$, $x = 1.5$.

2. **1** Removing the solution from the vial first prevents contaminating the remaining contents. There is potential for contaminating medication in the vial. If available, change to a filter needle before withdrawing medication from a vial. A vacuum is not created in a vial. Compatible medications may be mixed in the same syringe.

3. $\frac{0.4}{1} = \frac{0.2}{x}$, $0.4x = 0.2$, $x = \frac{0.2}{0.4}$, $x = 0.5$ mL.

4. **2** The ventrogluteal is easily found, not painful, and has no major nerves or blood vessels nearby.

   The deltoid is not always developed enough. The dorsogluteal is hard to find, has many injuries reported, is painful to lie on, and presents the possibility of sciatic nerve damage. The vastus lateralis may not be developed enough and may be more painful.

5. **1** The skin slides over to seal the medication in the muscle, preventing seepage of medications into the surrounding tissue. Aspiration should be performed, and Z-track diminishes but does not eliminate discomfort.

6. **1** Needles should not be recapped. Needleless devices are required, and recapping used needles needlessly exposes the nurse to bloodborne infections.

7. **2** Inserting and withdrawing the needle quickly decreases nerve ending stimulation and pain. Injecting slowly allows tissues time to separate and also decreases pain. Inserting and withdrawing the needle slowly causes pain, as does injecting quickly. Injecting quickly and withdrawing slowly both cause pain, and vigorous massage can damage tissue, causing more pain.

8. **4** The ventrogluteal site can be easily identified and reached in all of the above positions.

9. **1** A large-gauge needle (at least 20-gauge) is needed because this medication is thick.

10. **2** A small muscle will be adequate for this small volume of a medication. A large muscle (like vastus lateralis or ventrogluteal) is not needed. The dorsogluteal site is not recommended for IM injections.

11. Viscosity. You must choose a catheter gauge large enough to allow the medication to be injected easily.

12. Patient weight and injection site. You must choose a catheter long enough to reach the targeted muscle.

13. Parenteral. Refers to system that bypasses the gastrointestinal tract.

14. False. Avoid vigorous massage because it may cause tissue damage.

15. True. Change the needle to be sure no medication remains on the outside of the needle.

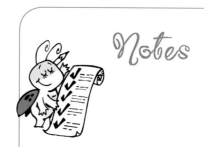

Notes

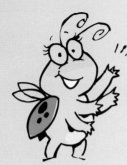

Chapter

7

Preparation and Administration of Powders

What You WILL LEARN

After reading this chapter, you will know how to do the following:

✔ Define powdered medication.
✔ Reconstitute medications supplied in powdered form.
✔ Calculate the amount of solute and solvent necessary to accurately prepare the medication as prescribed for the patient.

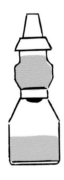

Because some medications lose their potency quickly in liquid form, they are prepared and shipped as powders. Before these medications are administered to patients, they must be converted to liquid form. This process is known as *reconstitution*. Reconstituted solutions may be administered orally (PO), or they can be given by intramuscular (IM), subcutaneous (SubQ), or intravenous (IV) injection. Once a powdered drug has been reconstituted, it has a limited shelf life. (You should consult the drug manufacturer's insert for information regarding shelf life and storage of reconstituted medications.)

What IS a Powdered Drug?

All *powdered drugs* are shipped in sealed vials or packages. If the medication is injectable, it is packaged in a sterile container and strict asepsis must be maintained as it is reconstituted. Some powdered drugs are accompanied by a special solution for mixing; however, most drugs may be safely mixed with sterile normal saline or sterile water (bacteriostatic with multidose vials). Oral medications usually (not always) are reconstituted with tap water. The liquid in which the drug is dissolved is called the *diluent*. The solution strength (concentration) resulting from the mixture of a powdered drug is the relationship of the powder to the diluent. The amount of medication is constant, but the volume of diluent may be changed. The more diluent added the less concentrated the solution. Some intravenous drugs come in use-activated systems with one compartment powder and the other the intravenous fluid bag. The user, at the time of administration, must activate the powder container and mix with the IV fluid (diluent) before administration. Special care must be taken to ensure that the medication compartment has been activated and has been thoroughly mixed with the IV fluid.

Although powdered drugs are sometimes reconstituted in the pharmacy, there are times when you will have to complete the reconstitution process before administration. Before the reconstitution process begins, check the preparation directions on the drug label or on the package insert. Remember that parenteral drug reconstitution requires you to use a strict aseptic technique (the drug and diluent are packaged as sterile items, and all needles and syringes used in reconstitution must also be sterile).

TAKE HOME POINTS

- Powdered drug + diluent = drug solution
- The amount of medication powder remains the same, but the volume diluent may be altered.
- 1 mL = 1 cc
- 1000 mg = 1 g

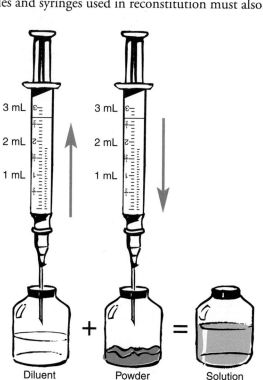

Diluent   +   Powder   =   Solution

What You NEED TO KNOW

- Always recheck the prescription before preparing a drug.
- Make sure the drug is in the correct form for its prescribed route of administration. For example, if a drug had been ordered for IM use, did you receive a drug that can be administered using the intramuscular route?
- Locate the directions for reconstitution on the drug label.
- Review the Six Rights of Medication Administration—the right drug, the right dose, the right patient, the right time, the right route, the right documentation (see Chapter 4).
- When reconstituting drugs, you should choose the correct diluent and the correct volume.

Penicillin G label.

On the above label, note that the vial contains 1 million Units. Because there are no conversion factors for units (they are specific to the particular drug), you cannot convert units to milligrams. According to the information provided on the drug label, you may prepare the drug in different strengths based on the volume of diluent you add. The following examples show how adding more diluent lessens the concentration of the solution:

Amount of Diluent Added	Concentration of Solution
1.6 mL	500,000 Units/mL
4.6 mL	200,000 Units/mL
9.6 mL	100,000 Units/mL

Note: The label does not specify a diluent solution. This suggests that a diluent solution accompanies the drug.

What You DO

To reconstitute a parenteral drug in powder form:

* Using strict aseptic technique and a sterile needle and syringe, add the appropriate volume of diluent to the powder.
* Mix the drug thoroughly by shaking or gently rolling the vial between your hands as directed by the manufacturer. Make sure all the powder is dissolved before administering the drug.
* Once the drug is reconstituted, you must specify the concentration (strength/volume) of the solution. Consider the previous example: If you add 4.6 mL of diluent, the resulting solution will contain 200,000 Units/mL.
* Keep in mind that the solution resulting from the powdered drug and diluent may be greater in volume than the solution added.
* Remember that once a drug has been reconstituted, it will lose its effectiveness after a given period of time (discard date). This time should be specified on the drug label, or the label should state, "Discard after _____ days."
* Write the date, time, the amount of diluent added, the concentration of solution, the discard date (if multidose), storage information (if not visible or label), and your initials on the reconstituted drug label.
* Store medication according to manufacturer's directions.

When a medication container is not properly labeled with date and time, the medication should be discarded and a new one used.

TAKE HOME POINTS

There are five basic points that you must consider when reconstituting medication:
1. Type of diluent to use
2. Volume of diluent to use
3. Concentration (strength/ volume) of the drug (after reconstitution)
4. Storage directions (after reconstitution)
5. Length of time drug is usable (after reconstitution)

Do You UNDERSTAND?

If any of the basic points are missing, consult the *Hospital Drug Formulary,* a pharmacology text; the *Physician's Desk Reference* (PDR); or the hospital pharmacy. You may also consult the Food and Drug Administration (FDA) web site at *www.fda.gov.*

DIRECTIONS: **Check the best answer.**

1. 10 mL + diluent powdered drug will provide a solution amount that is:
   a. _____ Less than the diluent
   b. _____ The same as the diluent
   c. _____ Greater than the diluent

Answers: 1. c.

2. According to the label on p. 112, adding 9.6 mL of sterile water to 1 million Units of Penicillin G will provide 100,000 Units per what?

   a. _____ ½ mL

   b. _____ 1.0 mL

   c. _____ 1.5 mL

   d. _____ 10.0 mL

3. Which key points should be remembered when reconstituting medication?

   a. _____ Patient's medical diagnosis

   b. _____ Medication order

   c. _____ Amount of diluent to be added

   d. _____ Strength of medication

   e. _____ Patient's financial status

   f. _____ Type of diluent to use

   g. _____ Immunization history

   h. _____ Storage of medication

   i. _____ Form of medication (IM or IV)

   j. _____ Patient's diet orders

   k. _____ Drug expiration date

What You NEED TO KNOW

After you have prepared and labeled a solution, it is time to focus on dose strength/volume. Consider the previous example in which 4.6 mL of diluent was added to a powdered drug to provide a concentration of 200,000 Units/mL. If you were asked to administer 250,000 Units, you would need to use the ratio and proportion method to calculate the correct dose. Remember that you DO NOT use the powdered drug or diluent volume in setting up your equation.

$$\frac{200{,}000 \text{ mL}}{1 \text{ mL}} = \frac{250{,}000 \text{ mL}}{x \text{ mL}}$$

- Cancel zeros and cross multiply.

$$20x = 25$$

- $x = \dfrac{25}{20}$ or $20\overline{)25.00}$ (1.25)

$x = 1.25$ mL to be administered.

Route of Administration

- If the medication is to be given IM, make sure that the amount of solution does not exceed the amount that can be safely injected.
- If the medication is to be given IM, make sure that the drug is sufficiently diluted so that the patient's tissues are not irritated.
- If the medication is to be given IV, remember that IV medications may require additional dilution after reconstitution and before administration.
- If the medication is to be given IV as a piggyback, intermittent, or continuous infusion, remember that the reconstituted drug will be added to an infusion bag (50 mL to 1000 mL).

Strength of Dose

When reconstituting a medication, choose a strength that comes closest to the amount prescribed. For example, the health care practitioner has prescribed 300,000 Units of Penicillin G, IM. You have a choice of adding 4.6 mL to provide 200,000 Units/mL; 9.6 mL to provide 100,000 Units/mL; or 1.6 mL to provide 500,000 Units/mL. Because 200,000 Units is closest to 300,000 Units, 4.6 mL would be the appropriate diluent volume to use.

Age-Specific Considerations

Pregnancy: During pregnancy, many drugs cross the placenta in minutes (particularly when they are administered IV). Most drugs that cross the placenta stabilize in the fetus at 50% to 100% of the maternal level. However, there also are drugs that have a higher rate of stabilization in the fetus than in the mother. Drugs are categorized by the Food and Drug Administration (FDA) *(www.fda.gov)* according to their safety when used during pregnancy.

FDA Pregnancy Categories

A. No risk is demonstrated to the fetus in any trimester.
B. No adverse effects are demonstrated in animals; no human studies are available.
C. Administered only after risks to the fetus are considered. Animal studies have shown adverse reactions; no human studies are available.
D. Definite fetal risks have been demonstrated. May be given despite risks if necessary in a life-threatening condition.
X. Will absolutely cause fetal abnormalities. Not to be used any time during pregnancy.

When working with a pregnant patient, you should consult the accompanying literature or pharmacology text to determine the safe use of any medication you are administering. Remember that the risk of a drug to a fetus is always weighed against the benefit of the drug to the mother.

Drugs Contraindicated During Pregnancy

Bromocriptine	Gold salts
Cimetidine	Methimazole
Clemastine	Methotrexate
Cyclophosphamide	Phenindione
Ergotamine	Thiouracil

Source: American Academy of Pediatrics Committee on Drugs.

Neonates: Because of varying percentages of total body water and immaturity of liver and kidney function, drugs must be carefully administered to premature infants and neonates. In addition, rapid changes in total body fluid and body weight may require frequent adjustment of drug doses.

Breast-fed infants: Certain drugs are contraindicated during breast-feeding (lactation). Transfer of drugs into breast milk is higher during the colostrum stage of milk production. In some instances, temporary discontinuation of breast-feeding may be advised.

Infancy and childhood: Medications are usually ordered for infants and children based on their weight and body surface area (BSA). BSA is considered the most accurate basis on which to calculate drug doses for children (see Chapter 2 for calculation of BSA). When administering medication to infants, remember that they have a body composition of approximately 75% water (adults have a body composition of 50% to 60% water).

Older adults: Drug absorption changes in individuals over 55 to 60 years of age. This is because body composition changes, with a decrease in total body water and muscle tissue and an increase in fatty tissue. Renal and hepatic clearance are also reduced during this stage of life. In addition, older adults often take multiple drugs that may interact with one another. Therefore standard adult medication doses may be excessive for older patients. You need to consider these factors when administering medications to older adults.

What You DO

- Check the patient's chart for allergies and other aversions to certain medications.
- Review your drug information card, text, or package insert for special points about the drug you are to administer.
- Review the Six Rights of Medication Administration: the right drug, the right dose, the right patient, the right date, the right time, and the right documentation.
- When reconstituting drugs, you should also consider the right diluent and the right volume.
- Prepare the medication.
- Ask the patient his or her name and verify it against the information provided on the patient's arm band.
- Assess the patient's general condition and ask about allergies.
- Explain the purpose of the medication and the route of administration.
- Administer medication.

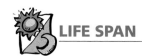

LIFE SPAN

- Calculation of drug dosages for infants and children are most accurately obtained based on body surface area (BSA).
- Drugs must be prescribed and administered with caution during pregnancy and lactation.
- Children have a *higher* percentage of total body water than adults.
- Older adults have a *lower* percentage of total body water than younger adults.

Do You UNDERSTAND?

DIRECTIONS: **Select the correct answer.**

1. You have added 8.5 mL of sterile water to 1 g (1000 mg) of penicillin to provide a solution in which 100 mg = 1 mL. Your order reads, "Give penicillin 250 mg intramuscular at 2 PM." How many milliliters will you need to provide a dose of 250 mg? Select the correct proportion to solve this problem:

   a. $\underline{\hspace{1cm}}$ $\dfrac{100 \text{ mg}}{1 \text{ mL}} = \dfrac{250 \text{ mg}}{x \text{ mL}}$

   b. $\underline{\hspace{1cm}}$ $\dfrac{1000 \text{ mg}}{1 \text{ mL}} = \dfrac{250 \text{ mg}}{8.5 \text{ mL}}$

   c. $\underline{\hspace{1cm}}$ $\dfrac{1000 \text{ mg}}{8.5 \text{ mL}} = \dfrac{250 \text{ mg}}{x \text{ mL}}$

2. How many milliliters will you give the patient? $\underline{\hspace{3cm}}$

Answers: 1. a; 2. 2.5 mL.

3. You have added 9.6 mL of diluent to 0.4 mL powdered penicillin G. The concentration is 100,000 Units/mL. How many milliliters will you give to provide the dose of 300,000 Units?

_____ mL

Penicillin G label.

4. Is this a safe amount of fluid to inject IM? _____
   If the medication order asks you to give 400,000 Units/dose, you add 1.6 mL diluent to provide a concentration of 500,000 Units/mL. *Remember that you should indicate the dose strength and expiration date of the reconstituted solution on the vial after reconstitution.*

5. If you reconstitute this drug at 1 PM on July 1 and refrigerate it, when should you discard it?
   a. _____ July 8 at 1 PM
   b. _____ July 3 at 1 PM
   c. _____ July 7 at 1 PM
   d. _____ July 2 at 12 AM

References

Curren AM, Munday LD: *Math for meds,* ed 9, San Diego, 2004, WI Publications.
Morris DG: *Calculate with confidence,* ed 3, St Louis, 2002, Mosby.
Skidmore-Roth L: *Mosby's drug guide for nurses,* St Louis, 2005, Mosby.

Answers: 3. 3; 4. Yes; 5. a.

NCLEX® Review

Refer to the oxacillin drug label when answering the following questions.

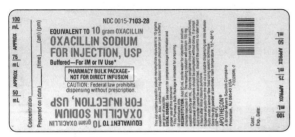

Oxacillin label.

1. Your patient has been prescribed 300 mg of oxacillin IM. You have a 500-mg vial of oxacillin in powdered form in stock. How much sterile water should you add to provide a dose of 250 mg/1.5 mL?
   1 1.5 mL
   2 10 mL
   3 2.7 mL
   4 3 mL

2. How many milliliters of Prostaphlin (oxacillin) will you give to obtain the prescribed dose of 300 mg?
   1 3 mL
   2 1.8 mL
   3 1.5 mL
   4 2 mL

3. Is this a safe amount to give IM?
   1 Yes
   2 No

4. Drugs must be used with caution in older adults because:
   1 They have a higher proportion of body fluid than younger adults.

2 They have a lower proportion of body fluid than younger adults.
   3 They have a lower proportion of fatty tissue than younger adults.
   4 They have a higher proportion of muscle tissue than younger adults.

5. The prescription for a young adult male is 400,000 Units Penicillin G intramuscular 4 times a day. Using label (see p. 118), what is the best volume of diluent to add?_____

Fill in the Blanks

6. Injectable medications require that you use _____ _____ when reconstituted.

7. A _____ is formed when a diluent is added to a powdered drug.

8. Concentration includes the _____ and _____ of the solution.

True or False

9. The main reason medications are prepared as powders is to take up less space.

10. When relabeling a drug after reconstitution, you need to include only the diluent added.

NCLEX® Review Answers

1. **3** You should add 2.7 mL of water to provide this dose, as stated on the label.

2. **2** Giving the patient 1.8 mL would provide the dose of 300 mg. Giving the patient 2 or 3 mL would be an excessive dose. Giving the patient 1.5 mL would be an inadequate dose.

3. **1** This is a safe amount (1.8 mL) to inject IM for an adult.

4. **2** Older adults have a *lower* proportion of body fluid than younger adults. Older adults have a *higher* proportion of fatty tissue and a *lower* proportion of muscle tissue than younger adults.

5. 1.6 mL. If a medication is to be given IM, make sure that the amount of solution does not exceed the amount that can be safely injected.

6. Aseptic technique. Asepsis must be maintained for every step of reconstitution with injectable medications.

7. Solution. A solution is the combination of a powdered drug plus the appropriate diluent.

8. Strength and volume. Concentration is the relationship of powdered drug to diluent. This is expressed as a ratio: strength/volume (milligrams/milliliter). The more diluent added, the less concentrated the solution; the less diluent added, the more concentrated the solution. The amount of diluent may be altered, but the amount of the powdered drug remains the same.

9. False. Some medications lose their potency in the liquid form.

10. False. When labeling a reconstituted drug, you should include the amount of diluent added, the concentration of the solution, the date of expiration, and your initials.

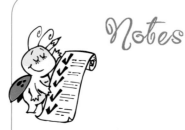

Notes

Administration of Subcutaneous and Intradermal Drugs

What You WILL LEARN

After reading this chapter, you will know how to do the following:

- ✔ Define a subcutaneous and an intradermal injection.
- ✔ Differentiate between medication types, dosages, and administration of subcutaneous and intradermal injections.
- ✔ Calculate appropriate amounts of prescribed medications for subcutaneous and intradermal injections.

Medications administered by injection may have local or systemic effects. By now you should be familiar with common injection methods (e.g., subcutaneous [SubQ, SC], intradermal [ID], intramuscular [IM], and intravenous [IV]). This chapter covers SubQ and ID injections.

What IS a Subcutaneous Injection?

A SubQ injection is given into the loose fat and connective tissue between the second layer of the skin and the muscle. Insulin, anticoagulants, colony-stimulating factors, and some vitamins are administered using this method.

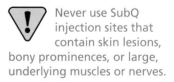 Never use SubQ injection sites that contain skin lesions, bony prominences, or large, underlying muscles or nerves.

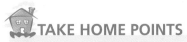

TAKE HOME POINTS

Because subcutaneous tissue contains pain receptors, only doses up to 1 mL of water soluble drugs should be given SubQ.

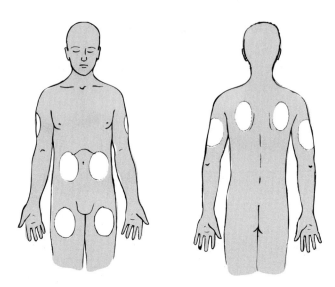

What You NEED TO KNOW

SubQ injection sites include the abdomen, below the edges of the last rib, and between the iliac crests; the outer posterior aspect of the upper arms; the fat pad over the insertion of the deltoid muscle in the upper arms; and the anterior aspects of the thigh. Less commonly used sites are the upper ventral or dorsal-gluteal areas of the buttocks and the shoulder blade areas of the upper back. Drugs injected SubQ are absorbed more slowly than drugs injected IM because the SubQ tissue is not as richly supplied with blood. Absorption from these sites is usually complete in patients with normal circulatory status; however, you should never use SubQ injection sites that contain skin lesions, bony prominences, or large, underlying muscles or nerves.

Drugs for SubQ injection may be packaged in a variety of ways: single-dose vials; multiple-dose vials; ampules; single-dose, prefilled cartridges; or ready-to-use, prefilled syringes. Needles come attached to syringes or may be packaged separately to allow for flexibility in gauge and length selection.

As you learned in Chapter 7, when adding diluent to a multiple-dose vial, you should write the date, the time, discard date, and your initials on the vial's label. Prefilled cartridges that require a plunger extension system (common types are Carpoject and Tubex) are used with their specific injection devices. The cartridge is mounted into the device, the air is usually cleared from the cartridge, and the injection is given in the usual manner. Directions for placing the cartridge into the injection device are supplied by the manufacturer and may be obtained from the pharmacy.

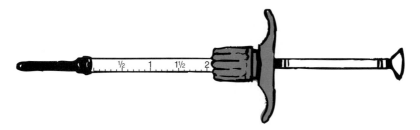

The depth of a patient's subcutaneous skin layer is indicated by his or her body weight; the more a person weighs, the more subcutaneous fat he or she is likely to have. However, when giving SubQ injections it is important to remember that fat distribution is influenced by sex and body shape, and that children and extremely underweight adults require shorter needles (³/8 to ⁵/8 inches) than do adults of average size. Also keep in mind that it may be necessary to insert the needle at a 45-degree angle when injecting small children and underweight adults.

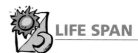

LIFE SPAN

Children and extremely underweight adults require shorter needles than do adults of average size. It may be necessary to insert the needle at a 45-degree angle when injecting small children and underweight adults.

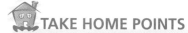

TAKE HOME POINTS

- For an overweight adult, pinch up the skin tissue and select a needle length of approximately one half the width of the skin fold.
- The higher the needle gauge number, the smaller the needle (for example, a 21-gauge needle has a bigger diameter than a 23-gauge needle).
- Since most drugs suitable for SubQ injections are water-soluble and not thick, they may be administered successfully with a 25- or 26-gauge needle.

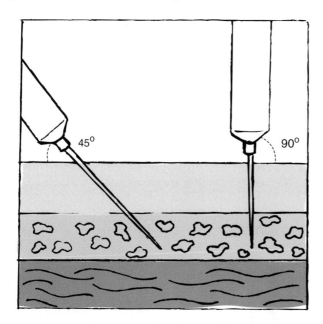

For an adult of above-average weight, you should pinch up the tissue and select a needle length that is approximately one half the width of the skin fold and an insertion angle that is between 45 and 90 degrees. Using this technique will ensure that the needle reaches the fatty tissue at the base of the skin fold.

Hypodermic, insulin, and tuberculin (TB) syringes may all be used to give SubQ injections. Hypodermic syringes come in a variety of sizes; the most commonly used for SubQ injections are 2.5- and 3-mL sizes.

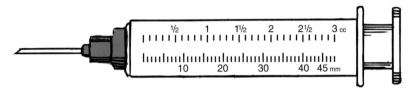

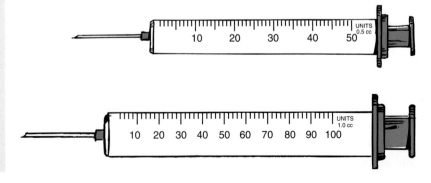

🏠 TAKE HOME POINTS

The unmarked calibration marks between numbered markings are commonly four. But the volume represented by these calibration markings is different depending on the size of the syringe.

Understanding the calibration marks on the syringe is critical to safely using syringes.

🏠 TAKE HOME POINTS

- When using an SubQ injection to administer insulin, use abdominal sites to ensure consistent absorption.
- When giving SubQ injections, avoid injecting a radius of 2 inches around the navel (injections may be more painful and absorption less reliable in this area).
- Each subsequent abdominal injection should be given at least 1 inch away from the previous one.
- Sites should be rotated so that a site is used only once a month to prevent the development of lipohypertrophy (i.e., spongy swelling) or lipoatrophy (i.e., loss of tissue leaving a depression) at the site.

Calibrations markings on syringes use the metric system. Syringes of 1 mL and 0.5 mL are calibrated in hundredths. Syringes of 2 mL, 2.5 mL, and 3 mL are calibrated in tenths. Larger syringes such as 5 mL, 6 mL, and 10 mL are calibrated in two-tenths increments. Syringes 20 mL and larger are calibrated in 1-mL increments. To prevent mistakes in measurement, you should select a syringe size based on the volume of drug to be drawn up.

Insulin syringes are used specifically for the administration of insulin. The syringes are calibrated in units and come in a low-dose sizes: 0.3 mL and 0.5 mL, and standard size 1 mL. When administering insulin, you should select a syringe size based on the dose of insulin being given. Because the calibration markings are so close and small on the 1-mL syringe, it is easier to correctly draw up low doses in the smaller syringes where the calibration markings are further apart. In the United States, insulin is only available in 100 units/mL. When giving insulin subcutaneously, keep in mind that the abdominal sites provide a faster, more consistent rate of absorption than other SubQ injection sites. For more about determining the dose of insulin, see Chapter 2.

What You DO

Because SubQ injections are given into tissue containing many pain receptors, administration techniques are very important. You can minimize discomfort to your patient by using a needle of the smallest suitable length and gauge. In addition, there are several things you need to consider when using this method of drug delivery:

- Follow routine procedure for withdrawing medication from a vial (see Chapter 6 for specific details).
- Cleanse the skin with alcohol and allow to dry.
- Hold the syringe like a dart, palm down, between the thumb and forefinger.
- For an average-size person, spread the skin tightly across the site or pinch up a skin fold with your nondominant hand. Inject the needle firmly and quickly at a 45- to 90-degree angle. If injecting an above-average weight person, pinch up a skin fold at the site and insert the needle at a 90-degree angle.
- Release the pinched skin before injecting the drug to avoid the discomfort of injecting a drug into compressed subcutaneous tissue. (Ignore this step when giving Lovenox.)
- Grasp the lower end of the syringe with your nondominant hand, and slowly, without moving the syringe, use your dominant hand to pull back on the plunger to aspirate the drug.
- If blood appears, withdraw the needle, discard the medication and syringe, and repeat the procedure (blood in the syringe indicates IV placement of the needle, which is undesirable for SubQ injections).
- If no blood appears, inject the drug slowly to minimize pain by allowing the subcutaneous tissue to separate gradually.
- When all of the drug is injected, withdraw the needle quickly and place an antiseptic swab or dry gauze over the site.

> ⚠ If blood appears, withdraw the needle, discard the medication and syringe, and repeat the procedure. Blood in the syringe indicates IV placement of the needle, which is undesirable for SubQ injections.
>
> When giving anticoagulants, such as heparin or Lovenox, do not massage the site after injection to prevent possible tissue damage and bleeding.

TAKE HOME POINTS

- In 1998, the American Diabetes Association issued a position statement explaining that when giving injections of insulin, routine aspiration is not necessary.
- Lovenox comes in prefilled syringes with specific administration directions that you should follow.
- Do not expel the air in a prefilled Lovenox syringe.
- Give Lovenox only in the lateral abdomen, with the patient lying down.
- When giving Lovenox, hold the skin pinch until all of the medication has been injected.
- For most other SubQ injections, aspiration is currently recommended. However, some authorities prefer not to aspirate. Therefore you should always be clear on the protocol used in your medical facility.

Do You UNDERSTAND?

DIRECTIONS: Unscramble the word or phrase in parentheses to fill in the blanks.

1. SubQ injections are given into loose fat and connective tissue between the second skin layer and the _____. *(eumslc)*
2. SubQ tissues contain _____ *(niap otcerpesr)* that limit the type and amount of drugs given SC.
3. SubQ injections should not be given in sites that have _____ _____ *(sink nisleos)*, or that are over _____ *(nyob sceiorpmnne)*.

DIRECTIONS: Label each statement *True* or *False*.

4. _____ Drugs for SubQ injection are only packaged in single- or multiple-dose vials.
5. _____ Prefilled cartridges are used with an injection device that allows injections to be given in the usual manner.
6. _____ Directions for using injection devices may be obtained from the facility pharmacy.
7. _____ After a multiple-dose vial has been opened, it must be labeled with the date and time, and you must sign it.
8. _____ SubQ injections may be given with hypodermic, insulin, and tuberculin syringes.
9. _____ Syringe size should be selected based on weight and age of the patient.
10. _____ To be used safely, insulin syringes must be marked to match the strength of insulin in units/mL.
11. _____ The abdomen is the site of choice for insulin administration because of its consistent rate of absorption.
12. _____ It is not necessary to rotate injection sites when giving insulin.

DIRECTIONS: **Match the following needle sizes and lengths with the appropriate person receiving a SubQ injection.**

13._____ 21 gauge, 1$^1\!/2$ inch a. Emaciated, older man
14._____ 25 gauge, $^5\!/8$ inch b. Not a good choice for SubQ injections
15._____ 26 gauge, $^3\!/8$ inch c. Slender, young woman

DIRECTIONS: **Check the appropriate measures you may take to minimize the pain associated with most SubQ injections.**

16. a. _____ Apply ice to the site.
 b. _____ Insert the needle quickly.
 c. _____ Inject the drug quickly.
 d. _____ Allow alcohol to dry before piercing the skin.
 e. _____ Inject the drug slowly.
 f. _____ Withdraw the needle quickly.
 g. _____ Release the pinched skin before injecting the drug.

DIRECTIONS: **When giving Lovenox, which of the chosen actions from question 16 should not be taken?**

17. _____

DIRECTIONS: **Complete the following statement.**

18. You may routinely aspirate most SubQ injections, except for
_____ and _____.

What IS an Intradermal Injection?

An *ID injection* is given into the dermis layer of the skin, just below the epidermis. Substances commonly administered in this manner include those used for allergy and TB skin testing. Because these solutions are very potent, injecting them ID provides a site where there is reduced blood supply and drug absorption can occur slowly. You can assess your patient's reaction to these substances by monitoring the degree of redness and swelling around the injection site.

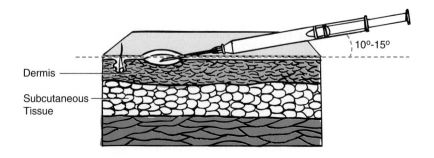

Dermis

Subcutaneous
Tissue

10°-15°

What You NEED TO KNOW

ID agents are injected just under the skin at a 10- to 15-degree angle. Sites for ID injection include the inside of the middle to upper forearm, the upper chest, and the upper back, just below the scapula (shoulder blade). Remember that doses given by ID injection are usually small (less than 0.5 mL).

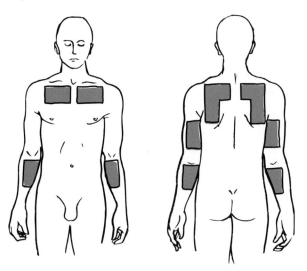

In both allergy and TB testing, you will use a TB syringe calibrated in tenths and hundreths of a millimeter. Needle size is usually 26 or 27 gauge and length is usually $^3/_8$ to $^5/_8$ inches. In allergy testing, 0.02 mL of a 1:1000 or 1:1500 concentration of test extract is injected.

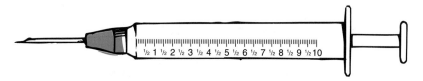

For comparison purposes, a control solution is also injected. A wheal (i.e., bump) that appears within 15 minutes of the injection and is 0.5 cm or larger than the control wheal is considered a positive reaction. Large skin reactions are often accompanied by physical symptoms, such as coughing, wheezing, itching, and rash.

TB testing is done by injecting tuberculin units ID. The tuberculin unit is the standard unit of measurement for the purified protein derivative (PPD) of TB. The standard dose is 5 tuberculin units in 0.1 mL of solution (Nasrawi and Allender, 1999). Between 48 and 72 hours after injection, the test is read (usually by a health care practitioner in the clinic in which it was administered). The area should be lightly rubbed from the area of normal skin to the indurated (i.e., hardened) area. Next the indurated area should be circled with a pencil and measured. Palpable induration (i.e., hardness, not redness) of more than 5 mm after 48 hours is considered a positive reaction.

Age-Specific Considerations

When testing certain age groups for allergies or TB, there are several things that you should consider:

Children: Allergy testing is frequently performed on young children. To decrease the child's anxiety, the least invasive methods should be used. The skin prick method (i.e., pricking the skin without causing bleeding) is preferable to the ID injection method.

Pregnant and lactating women: Pregnant and lactating women should check with their obstetrician or pediatrician before undergoing allergy or TB testing.

Older adults: Because their immune systems are less responsive than younger persons, older adults may have false-negative reactions to TB tests. Therefore older patients with known exposure to TB should have chest x-ray studies.

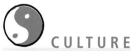

CULTURE

Redness may be present, particularly in light-skinned persons. However, in dark-skinned persons it may not be apparent. Check agency policy for follow-up based on degree of reaction. A chest x-ray film is necessary with all positive reactions.

After receiving an allergy injection, the patient should be closely observed for reactions, such as itching, wheezing, coughing, and possible anaphylactic shock. Emergency drugs, including epinephrine and Benadryl, and equipment for intubation should be on hand in the event of a negative reaction.

TAKE HOME POINTS

- ID solutions are injected just under the skin at a 10- to 15-degree angle.
- ID injections should always be administered with a TB syringe to ensure accuracy of dose.
- Properly injected solutions will cause a small wheal to appear at the injection site.

What You DO

Because of the nature of ID preparations, their administration requires great accuracy and care:

- Solutions are administered using a 1-mL tuberculin syringe calibrated in hundredths of a millimeter.
- You should follow the procedure for withdrawing medication from a vial (see Chapter 6).
- Cleanse the skin with alcohol and allow to dry before injecting the preparation.
- To allow easier piercing of skin, use your nondominant hand to stretch the skin over the site.
- With the bevel up and the needle almost against the patient's skin, insert the needle at a 10- to 15-degree angle, about $^1/_8$ inch below the skin surface.
- Inject the solution slowly, watching for the appearance of wheal or small blister (it is normal to feel resistance at this point).
- Withdraw the needle quickly and swab gently with alcohol (do not massage the site).

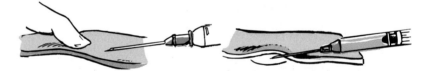

Do You UNDERSTAND?

DIRECTIONS: **Match the terms in Column A with the appropriate statements in Column B.**

Column A

1. _____ Induration
2. _____ 0.1 mL of solution
3. _____ 0.02 mL of 1:1000 injection strength solution
4. _____ Redness
5. _____ ½ inch
6. _____ ¾ inch

Column B

a. Appropriate needle length for ID injection
b. May be present if TB test is positive
c. Inappropriate needle length for ID
d. Standard dose for TB test
e. Must be present if TB test is positive
f. Usual dose for allergy testing

DIRECTIONS: **Place a check next to the key point that indicates a positive TB test.**

7. a. _____ Redness is present at more than 10 mm.
   b. _____ Induration occurs at greater than 5 mm.
   c. _____ Induration is greater than 3 mm.
   d. _____ Redness is greater than 5 mm.

DIRECTIONS: **Select the best answer.**

8. What is the standard dose for TB testing?
   a. _____ 1.0 mL
   b. _____ 0.1 mL
   c. _____ 0.001 mL
   d. _____ 10.0 mL

References

American Diabetes Association: Position statement: insulin administration, *Diabetes Care* 21(suppl 1):S72, 1998.

Chernecky C, Berger BJ: *Laboratory tests and diagnostic procedures,* ed 3, Philadelphia, 2004, WB Saunders.

Harkreader H: *Fundamentals of nursing: caring and clinical judgment,* Philadelphia, 2000, WB Saunders.

Kee JL, Hayes ER: *Pharmacology: a nursing process approach,* ed 2, Philadelphia, 1997, WB Saunders.

Lindeman CA, McAthie M: *Fundamentals of contemporary nursing practice,* Philadelphia, 1999, WB Saunders.

Macklin D, Chernecky C, Infortuna H: *Math for clinical practice,* St. Louis, 2005, Mosby.

Morris DG: *Calculate with confidence,* ed 3, St Louis, 2002, Mosby.

Nasrawi C, Allender J: *Quick and easy dosage calculations,* Philadelphia, 1999, WB Saunders.

Poland GA et al: Determination of deltoid fat pad thickness: implications for needle length in adult immunizations, *JAMA* 277:1709, 1997.

Potter PA, Perry AG: *Basic nursing: a critical thinking approach,* ed 2, St Louis, 1999, Mosby.

Skidmore-Roth L: *Mosby's drug guide for nurses,* St Louis, 2005, Mosby.

NCLEX® Review

Circle the correct answer.

1. Drugs injected SubQ are usually absorbed more slowly than drugs injected IM because:
   1 They are not as viscous as drugs injected IM.
   2 The subcutaneous tissue has less blood supply than muscle tissue.
   3 The subcutaneous tissue contains pain receptors.
   4 They contain preservatives that inhibit absorption.

2. When selecting a needle for an SubQ injection, you must consider the fact that the heavier your patient is:
   1 The larger the needle gauge should be
   2 The shorter the needle length should be
   3 The longer the needle length should be
   4 The smaller the needle gauge should be

3. When injecting heparin SubQ, you should remember:
   1 To massage the site afterward
   2 To insert the needle slowly
   3 To prevent pinching up the skin
   4 To prevent aspirating before injecting

4. When giving insulin, abdominal sites:
   1 May be used without rotating because absorption is consistent over time
   2 Should include the area directly around the navel because it is not as sensitive to pain
   3 Should be rotated to prevent lipohypertrophy or lipoatrophy
   4 Should not be used because they have a slower rate of absorption than other SubQ sites

5. You are instructing a patient in how to give her daily SubQ injections of insulin. According to the American Diabetes Association's new recommendations, you should teach her to avoid:
   1 Drawing back on the plunger before injecting her insulin
   2 Using the abdominal SubQ injection sites
   3 Using alcohol sponges to clean the area
   4 Rotating sites used in the abdominal area

6. Emergency drugs and equipment should be available in allergy clinics because:
   1 Persons with allergies are more likely to have heart attacks.
   2 Persons undergoing allergy testing are often very ill.
   3 Anaphylactic reactions sometimes occur with allergy testing.
   4 Persons administering allergy solutions often make errors.

7. Intradermal (ID) medications should be administered at an angle of which degree:
   1 45
   2 90
   3 30
   4 15

8. Which of the following is considered a positive reaction in intradermal tuberculosis testing?
   1 More than 12 mm of reddened area is observed.
   2 Induration is present at greater than 3 mm.
   3 Induration is present at greater than 10 mm.
   4 Redness is greater than 5 mm.

9. A major advantage of ID injection is that:
   1 It is the least painful injection method.
   2 Medication is more rapidly absorbed than when given with SubQ or IM injections.

3 The blood supply to this area is reduced, and the drug is absorbed more slowly.

4 Children will be more cooperative with this method.

Fill in the Blanks

10. Tuberculin syringes are calibrated in _____

11. Insulin syringes are calibrated in _____

12. 3 mL syringes are calibrated in _____

13. In the United States, insulin is only available in

_____

True or False

14. SubQ injections are less painful than other types of injections.

15. The subcutaneous route is the best choice for TB testing.

NCLEX® Review Answers

1. **2** Fewer blood vessels means slower absorption. Less viscosity would generally increase absorption rate. Pain receptors do not influence absorption, and most drugs given subcutaneously do not contain preservatives or other substances that inhibit absorption.

2. **3** The needle should be long enough to penetrate the SubQ tissue but not long enough to reach the underlying muscle. Needle diameter is not determined by body weight. A shorter needle would not penetrate to the SubQ layer in an overweight person. Selection of needle gauge is not based on body weight.

3. **4** Avoiding aspiration before injecting prevents trauma. Massaging the site after SubQ injection causes bruising. To minimize pain, insert the needle quickly, and pinch up the skin to allow for deep SubQ injection without injecting into the muscle.

4. **3** Rotating sides prevents these conditions. Absorption may be adversely affected by using the same site repeatedly. The area directly around the navel may be more painful to use, but absorption rates are timely and consistent at the abdominal sites.

5. **1** Drawing back the plunger before injecting her insulin is not necessary for routine insulin injections. Abdominal subcutaneous sites are excellent sites for injecting insulin. Use of alcohol swabs decreases the chance of infection, and rotation of sites is necessary to prevent lipohypertrophy and lipoatrophy.

6. **3** Anaphylaxis may occur if the patient has a positive reaction to a test injection. Persons with allergies are not more prone to heart attack, and perfectly healthy people undergo allergy testing. Many precautions are taken to prevent errors.

7. **4** ID injections are optimal if given at an angle between 15 and 20 degrees. SubQ, not ID, injections are given at an angle between 45 and 90 degrees.

8. **3** Any induration of 5 mm or more is an indication of a positive reaction in TB testing. Redness may occur over the testing area, but it is not an indication of a positive reaction. An induration of 3 mm is too small to determine a positive response to TB testing.

9. **3** ID injections allow potent medications to be absorbed over time. Pain is not a factor in the use of ID injections, but medication is more rapidly absorbed in SubQ injections. When giving injections to children, their cooperation is difficult to predict.

10.   hundredths.

11.   units.

12.   tenths.

13.   100 Units/mL.

14.   False. SubQ injections may be more painful because of the many pain receptors.

15.   False. Intradermal technique is used for TB testing.

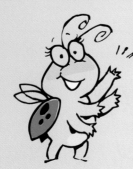

Chapter 9

Measurement and Administration of Topical Medications

What You WILL LEARN

After reading this chapter, you will know how to do the following:
- ✔ Define topical medication.
- ✔ Recognize and select the appropriate amount of topical medication to administer based on patient's prescription

Topical medications come in various forms. Although most topical medications produce a local effect (i.e., they affect the application area), others produce a systemic effect (i.e., they affect body systems). As a health care provider, you must be familiar with various forms of topical medications and their possible side effects.

What IS a Topical Medication?

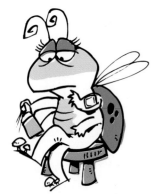

A *topical medication* is a preparation that is applied to the surface of the body. In some cases, topical medications may also be applied into body cavities or orifices, such as the eyes and ears (see Chapter 10) or the vagina and rectum (see Chapter 11).

Examples of topical medications include acne medications, used to reduce blemishes; glucocorticoids, used to decrease inflammation and itching; keratolytic agents, used to promote shedding of the outer cells of the skin; débriding enzymes, used to remove foreign material and necrotic tissue; vasodilators and vasoconstrictors, used to alter blood flow to the skin or to internal organs; local anesthetics, used to relieve pain or provide local anesthesia; local antiinfective agents, used to prevent or treat infection; and ectoparasiticides, used to kill mites and lice. All these medications may be applied directly to the skin or mucous membranes. Topical anesthetics are applied directly to the area that is to be desensitized.

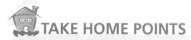

TAKE HOME POINTS

Always check to ensure that patients can swallow before allowing them to eat or drink after they have received topical anesthesia for diagnostic procedures, such as a bronchoscopy or laryngoscopy.

What You NEED TO KNOW

Most topical medications are locally acting and produce few side effects. In addition, the vehicle or type of topical preparation may actually provide extra benefits by acting as a moisturizer or drying agent. However, it is important to keep in mind that some topical medications given by metered dose inhalation (MDI) or transdermal patches are considered sympathomimetic agents (adrenergic drugs), and they may cause adverse reactions in your patients. Nitroglycerin (NTG), estrogen, and duragesic are commonly given by transdermal patch. (The essentials of using transdermal patches, including NTG and duragesic patches, are discussed in Chapter 14.)

Topical medications come in various forms:

Creams: Water-based, semisolid preparations

Gels: Translucent or clear, semisolid preparations that liquefy on contact with the skin

Lotions: Emollient liquid solutions, emulsions, or suspensions (may be oil- or water-based)

Ointments: Semisolid drug preparations, usually oil-based, that penetrate the skin better than a paste

Pastes: Semisolid preparations with adhesive properties (pastes are thicker than ointments or creams)

Patches: Adhesive materials with medication in the center (patches allow for secure placement and absorption of medication through the skin over extended periods)

Powder: Finely ground drugs that are sprinkled on the skin surface

Sprays: Liquids dispensed in fine droplets from a small bottle or inhaler

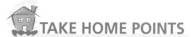

TAKE HOME POINTS

Topical preparations may be messy and may stain or leave a residue on clothing. Topical nerve growth factor is effective in treating severe, noninfected, pressure ulcers of the foot.

Topical Vitamin D analog, calciprotriene, is effective in treating plaque psoriasis. Accutane (Isotretinoin), a treatment for *acne vulgaris* in adolescents, has reported side effects of depression, psychosis, and rarely suicidal ideation.

Age-Specific Considerations

Adults: When treating patients with pubic lice, their sexual partners should be treated at the same time to avoid reinfestation. When using Retin-A (Tretinoin) and Adapalene to treat acne or remove fine wrinkles, remember that these drugs increase susceptibility to sunburn. You should remind your patients to wear sunscreen and protective clothing and avoid using these medications on individuals with existing sunburn.

Children: When treating children with scabies (i.e., mites) or pediculosis (i.e., lice), remind parents to wash and dry bedding and clothing at hot temperatures to prevent reinfestation. To prevent spreading head lice, children should also avoid sharing hats, combs, or brushes. Infants being treated with glucocorticosteroids in the diaper area should not wear disposable, plastic-lined diapers or plastic pants because they act as an occlusive dressing (i.e., a dressing that seals the wound completely). Instead the child should wear cloth diapers or training pants without plastic covers.

What You DO

- Use water to wash the affected area, and pat it dry before applying topical medications (unless the prescription directs otherwise).
- Shake lotions before using to distribute suspended particles. Use sterile gauze to pat lotions onto the affected area (rubbing may irritate the area).
- Apply ointments, creams, and pastes with gloves or a tongue depressor, and spread a thin layer over the affected area.
- Use a sterile dressing, if desired, after applying most ointments. Unless it has been prescribed, do not use an occlusive dressing over a corticosteroid ointment or cream (it may increase absorption through the skin and increase the possibility of systemic effects).
- When applying a transdermal patch, remove any drug residue from the former site before placing the next patch.
- To prevent skin irritation, rotate the sites where transdermal patches are used.
- Before applying débriding enzymes to remove necrotic tissue or foreign material, be sure to remove detergent or antiseptic compounds from an area. These compounds may inactivate enzyme action.

TAKE HOME POINTS

After receiving topical preparations for the treatment of scabies (mites) or pediculosis (lice), patients should be instructed to machine wash and dry all bedding and clothing at hot temperatures to prevent reinfestation.

Always wear gloves, or use tongue depressors or sterile swabs, to apply topical medications to prevent medicating yourself.

Check the affected site for broken skin. Applying drugs to broken skin could cause them to be absorbed rapidly, causing systemic effects.

When applying a débriding agent, avoid surrounding healthy skin or bright pink granulation tissue.

Follow exact directions for applying topicals to prevent administering too much or too little of the drug. Keep in mind that the potency of a topical drug is affected not only by the concentration, but by the natural activity of the drug, the vehicle used, and the method of application.

- Determine the dose of medication to be administered. (If an ointment, cream, or paste is packaged in a tube, often the dose will be measured by the length of the medication squeezed from the tube. A guide is usually provided with the product to assist in determining the required dose.)

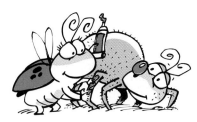

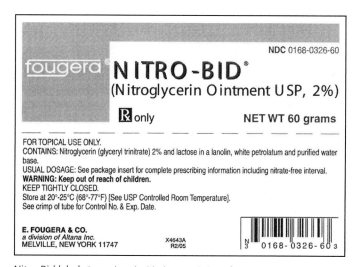

NDC 0168-0326-60

NITRO-BID®
(Nitroglycerin Ointment USP, 2%)

℞ only   NET WT 60 grams

FOR TOPICAL USE ONLY.
CONTAINS: Nitroglycerin (glyceryl trinitrate) 2% and lactose in a lanolin, white petrolatum and purified water base.
USUAL DOSAGE: See package insert for complete prescribing information including nitrate-free interval.
WARNING: Keep out of reach of children.
KEEP TIGHTLY CLOSED.
Store at 20°-25°C (68°-77°F) [See USP Controlled Room Temperature].
See crimp of tube for Control No. & Exp. Date.

E. FOUGERA & CO.
a division of Altana Inc.
MELVILLE, NEW YORK 11747   X4643A
                                  R2/05

N3   0168-0326-60 3

Nitro-Bid label. *Reproduced with the permission of E. Fougera and Co.*

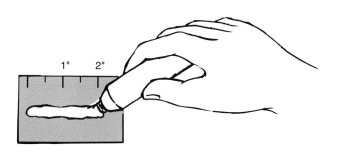

1"   2"

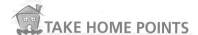

TAKE HOME POINTS

- Warm ointments, creams, and pastes by rubbing your gloved hands together.
- If your patients have an aversion to the smell of certain topical medications, have them suck on a peppermint or distract them while applying it.

⚠ If a medication causes a burning sensation, assure your patient that it will last for only a moment. If the burning sensation persists, remove the medication, document the problem, and contact the prescribing professional.

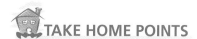

TAKE HOME POINTS

Topical preparations commonly contain more than one type of drug. Therefore you must determine if your patient has allergies to any of the drugs contained in a particular medication before applying it.

- Explain to patients who have been prescribed transdermal patches how they can calculate the exact time to remove and replace patches to ensure optimal drug effectiveness. For example: A health care practitioner has prescribed an Estraderm 0.025 mg/day patch twice weekly, and your patient applied her first patch at 8 PM on Monday evening.

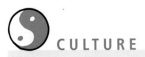

CULTURE

Tattoos may obscure local allergic reactions to some topical medications.

To determine when she should apply the second patch, you would need to use the following formula:

$$\frac{7 \text{ days}}{\text{week}} \times \frac{\text{week}}{2 \text{ doses}} = \frac{7}{2} = 3.5 \text{ days to next dose}$$

3.5 days from 8 PM Monday to 8 AM Friday

- Return an hour after administering any topical medication to evaluate for side effects and to document your related nursing interventions.

Do You UNDERSTAND?

DIRECTIONS: **Match the following terms in Column A with the descriptions in Column B.**

Column A	Column B
1. _____Ointment	a. Semisolid preparation with adhesive properties; thicker than ointments or creams
2. _____Patch	b. Drug sprinkled on the skin surface
3. _____Gel	c. Oil-based semisolid that penetrates skin well
4. _____Lotion	d. Water-based, semisolid preparation
5. _____Paste	e. Adhesive material with medication in the center; used for extended absorption
6. _____Powder	f. Clear semisolid that liquifies on contact with the skin
7. _____Cream	g. Emollient liquids, emulsions, or suspensions; either oil- or water-based

DIRECTIONS: **Label each statement *True* or *False*.**

8. _____ There are many medications that can be given topically.

9. _____ Topical medications may have systemic or local effects.

10. _____ Topical medications may be applied to the skin or into body cavities, eyes, or ears.

11. _____ Anesthetics are not used topically.

12. _____ Inhaled medications are not considered topical.

Answers: 1. c; 2. e; 3. f; 4. g; 5. a; 6. b; 7. d; 8. True; 9. True; 10. True; 11. False; 12. False.

DIRECTIONS: Unscramble the word or phrase in parentheses to fill in the blanks.

13. Abrasions may cause _____ absorption of topically applied drugs, resulting in systemic effects. *(dipar)*

14. Topical medications may stain or leave a _____ on clothes. *(edurise)*

15. Before applying most topical medications, _____ and dry the area. *(haws)*

16. To distribute suspended particles, always _____ lotions before using them. *(haske)*

17. Using sterile gauze, apply lotions by _____ them onto the affected area. *(tapntig)*

18. Do not clap your hands, but _____ them together to warm creams, ointments, or pastes. *(ubr)*

19. Ointments, pastes, and creams should be applied in a _____ layer over the affected area. *(htni)*

References

Kieffer MA. Pharmacology review. Topical vitamin D analogs, *Dermatol Nurs* 16(1): 89-90, 93, 100, 2004.

Landi F, Aloe L, Russo A et al: Topical treatment of pressure ulcers with nerve growth factor: a randomized clinical trial, *Ann Intern Med* 139(8):651-4, I-10, 2003.

Lerman C, Kaufmann V, Rukstalis M et al: Individualizing nicotine replacement therapy for the treatment of tobacco dependence: a randomized trial, *Ann Intern Med* 140(6):426-33, I-47, 2004.

Topical steroids. *Nurs Pract Prescribing Reference* 10(4):92, 2003.

Answers: **13.** rapid; **14.** residue; **15.** wash; **16.** shake; **17.** patting; **18.** rub; **19.** thin.

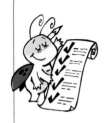

Notes

NCLEX® Review

Circle the correct answer.

1. Topical medications:
   1 Never cause systemic effects
   2 Are usually applied only to the skin
   3 May have systemic effects or local effects
   4 Have no side effects

2. Jan Cramer has Retin A Gel 0.01% prescribed for her acne. Which of the following should you instruct her to do?
   1 Wear sunscreen and protective clothing to prevent sunburn.
   2 Use a drying soap on her face each morning and evening.
   3 Eat peanuts and other legumes.
   4 Use no makeup until the course of treatment is finished.

3. Sara Svenson is a toddler receiving desoximetasone (Topicort) for a rash in the diaper area. As the health care practitioner, you should instruct her mother to:
   1 Change her plastic-lined, disposable diapers more frequently.
   2 Use sterile diapers from a diaper service and plastic pants.
   3 Use cloth diapers without plastic pants.
   4 Start using disposable, pull-up diapers for toddlers.

4. You have been asked to administer a thin layer of Travase cream (a débriding enzyme preparation) followed by application of a wet to dry dressing to a decubitus ulcer on your patient's right heel. You should apply the cream:
   1 Before your patient's whirlpool treatment
   2 In a patting motion
   3 Liberally, with a 4 × 4 gauze pad
   4 Using sterile gloves or a tongue blade

5. Mrs. Tomberlin is using an over-the-counter corticosteroid cream to decrease the itching associated with an outbreak of poison ivy on several areas of her body. She calls to ask you if she may cover the medicated areas with waterproof bandages so they won't look so bad. You should advise her:
   1 That if she covers the areas with any type of dressing, they will become further inflamed
   2 That absorption of the drug may increase significantly if she covers the area with a waterproof dressing, and systemic effects may result
   3 That she may use any type of dressing she wishes because absorption of corticosteroids is not affected by the type of dressing used
   4 That the plastic used in the manufacture of waterproof bandages interacts with corticosteroids to produce systemic reactions

6. You are wearing sterile gloves and applying an emollient cream to your patient's back. To warm the cream, you should:
   1 Put it in the microwave for 15 seconds.
   2 Palpate the tube vigorously.
   3 Run hot water over the cream.
   4 Rub your gloved hands together.

7. The health care practitioner prescribes Mycitracin Plus ointment, containing bacitracin, neomycin, polymyxin B, and lidocaine for a patient with an infected ingrown toenail. You know you have taken the proper precautions and instructed your patient to use the medication correctly if he or she states:
   1 "I am not allergic to any of the drugs listed on the label."
   2 "I will not use a bandage over this medicine."
   3 "I don't need to wash the old ointment off before applying the new ointment."
   4 "This ointment won't leave a residue on anything."

8. Applying topical medications to abrasions may result in:
   1 Allergic reactions
   2 Increased absorption and systemic effects
   3 Increased healing time
   4 Necrotic tissue development

9. When administering a débriding enzyme preparation, you should avoid applying the cream to:
   1 The center of a necrotic lesion
   2 The bright pink tissue at the edge of the lesion
   3 The darker tissue at the edge of a lesion
   4 The blanched tissue with exudate

10. A transdermal patch is a popular way to deliver a topical drug that has:
    1 A short-lived effect
    2 No systemic effect
    3 A prolonged effect
    4 A local effect

11. True or False? Topical medications that affect only the application area are known as systemic medications that produce systemic effects.

12. Fill in the blank. Topical medications used to remove foreign material and necrotic tissue are known as _____ enzymes.

13. Short answer: What is the categorical name of agents used to relieve local pain or provide local numbness or local lack of feeling? Local _____

14. Short answer: Your patient has just undergone a bronchoscopy 2 hours ago. The patient is prescribed a pain pill he has been known to take to help relieve pain in the past. The patient states he now has pain. What assessment is necessary before you administer the pain pill? _____

15. Short answer: Your patient is prescribed a fentanyl (Duragesic) patch, 25 mcg/hour, every 72 hours for pain control. The patch was placed on his torso Friday at 10 AM (1000 hours). When is the next patch due to be administered? _____

NCLEX® Review Answers

1. **3** If topical medications are applied by transdermal patch or inhaled, they have systemic effects. Topical medications are sometimes applied in body cavities and mucous membranes. All medications can potentially have side effects.

2. **1** Retin A increases susceptibility to sunburn. Dry skin may result from Retin A, and you don't want to aggravate it with a drying soap. Eating peanuts and legumes has nothing to do with Retin A side effects, and cosmetics may be used while undergoing treatment with Retin A.

3. **3** Air flow is not occluded, and increased absorption will not result. Plastic pants act as an occlusive dressing. Plastic liners used with disposable pull-up diapers also act as occlusive dressings.

4. **4** Using sterile gloves or a tongue blade prevents self-medication. Applying the cream before a whirlpool treatment allows it to wash off. A thin, even layer is necessary, and a 4 × 4 gauze pad may not protect your hands.

5. **2** Corticosteroid absorption may increase and systemic effects result if occlusive dressings are used. A dressing itself does not cause inflammation. Absorption is affected by type of dressing. There is no interaction between the plastic and corticosteroid drugs.

6. **4** Rubbing the cream between gloved hands will warm it to body temperature. Never use a microwave to warm cream because it may become too hot. Palpation will not affect temperature of the cream in the tube. Hot water may dissolve or remove the cream from your gloves.

7. **1** Topicals may contain several drugs. You must be sure the patient is not allergic to any of them. A bandage may be used. Your patient should remove any remaining ointment before applying new ointment, and ointments may leave residue or stains on clothing or other material.

8. **2** Abrasions or denuded skin may allow more rapid absorption of the medication and result in unintended systemic effects. Applying topicals to an abrasion will not cause an allergic reaction unless a patient is allergic to the drug, but topicals may actually decrease healing time. Applying topicals to abraded areas does not result in development of necrosis.

9. **2** Bright pink tissue is healthy granulation tissue; you do not want to break it down. Débriding enzyme should be applied to all necrotic tissue in a lesion (including darker tissue at the edge of a lesion). Enzyme action will clean out the dead cells and exudate.

10. **3** Transdermal patches are frequently used to deliver drugs in a form that provides a prolonged effect. They are usually used for systemic effects.

11. False. Affected area–only medications are known as local effect medications.

12. débriding.

13. anesthetics.

14. Assess the swallowing reflex/ability to prevent aspiration/harm.

15. Monday 10 AM or Monday 1000 hours.

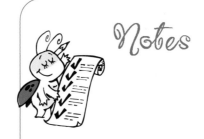

Notes

Eye, Ear, and Nose Medications

10

What You WILL LEARN

After reading this chapter, you will know how to do the following:

✔ Differentiate medication types, dosages, and methods of administration of eye, ear, and nose medications.

✔ Determine the correct dose of eye and ear medications based on availability and prescription.

Most eye, ear, and nose drugs are instilled directly into the applicable body cavity in the form of drops, ointments, or sprays. Anesthetics and drugs used to treat inflammation; bacterial, fungal, and viral infections; and other diseases are supplied in unit-dose or monodrop containers that dispense one drop at a time. This chapter covers the essentials of measuring and administering eye, ear, and nose medications.

What IS an Eye Medication?

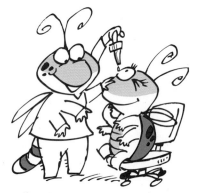

Eye medications are NEVER placed directly onto the cornea

Eye medications come in the form of drops, ointments, and medicated discs. Because the cornea is richly supplied with pain fibers and is very sensitive, eye medications are NEVER placed directly onto the cornea. Instead, they are placed in the conjunctival sac (i.e., lower lid).

You should advise your patients who wear contact lenses to substitute glasses for the duration of treatment with eye drops, ointments, or discs, unless the product specifically states that it is formulated to be used with contact lenses.

What You NEED TO KNOW

Eye drops are usually packaged in monodrop plastic containers that allow one drop at a time to be administered. If a separate dropper is provided, you should only use that dropper to administer the medication. Use of another dropper may cause an overdose or underdose of the drug.

Frequently, abbreviations are used to identify the eye for which a drug is intended: OD indicates the right eye, OS indicates the left eye, and OU indicates both eyes. You should always verify the abbreviations used by your institution. To ensure accuracy, also verify the meaning of any abbreviation written by the prescribing health care professional if it is unclear to you.

When administering eye drops, you must be sure that the drops are the same size. To do this, hold the dropper or container perpendicular to the inside of the conjunctival sac so that the drop hangs freely, then drops off. When more than one drop is to be given, wait 5 minutes between drops. This ensures that the original drop is not washed away by the second drop, or that the second drop is not diluted by the first.

You should teach your patients to discard any discolored or darkened solutions. Most eye drops have a 90-day shelf life or, once opened, they may be used to the end of the current illness. When not in use, the container should be closed tightly to prevent contamination and stored as directed on the label.

Systemic absorption of eye drops can cause adverse reactions, especially if an interaction occurs between the drug given as an eye drop and a drug taken by another route. For example, timolol, a beta blocker given to decrease intraocular pressure, may interact with oral beta blockers to cause additive bradycardia. Timolol may also interact with organophosphate insecticides or pesticides, and cardiovascular and respiratory arrest may result.

Ophthalmic ointments are usually contained in very small tubes. Prescribed strengths for ophthalmic drugs are usually dilute (i.e., less than 1% concentration). When ocular ointments are used for the first

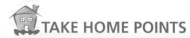

TAKE HOME POINTS

Always check to be sure that any drug used in the eye is labeled for ophthalmic use only and is in a sterile package.

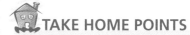

TAKE HOME POINTS

Abbreviations should be written out to avoid errors.

TAKE HOME POINTS

To decrease the risk of transmitting an infection from one eye to the other, do not touch the eyelids, lashes, or other structures with eye droppers or ointment tubes. Drug containers for optic (eye) and otic (ear) preparations look very similar, so you must be sure that medications to be used in the eye are labeled for *optic* or *ophthalmic* use.

Do not dose the unaffected eye. Explain to the patient that he or she should never allow a person to use his or her eye medicine. Injury or allergic reaction could result.

time, the first $^1/_4$ inch should be discarded to ensure sterility of the drug. If the patient has more than one ocular drug preparation to be given at the same time, wait 5 minutes after placing the ointment before giving drops (wait 10 minutes if the patient is to have another ointment).

Intraocular discs are medicated discs that look like contact lenses. They are placed in the conjunctival sac on the sclera between the iris and lower eyelid, and may remain in place for up to 1 week. You should teach your patients who have been prescribed intraocular discs to report any itching, pain, or swelling (it may indicate an adverse reaction to the drug or disc).

What You DO

Many adverse effects have been reported when a patient wearing contact lenses takes certain oral medications or applies a topical medication to the eyes. Soft lenses may enhance the pharmacologic effects of eye drops or ointments by absorbing the medication and releasing it over time. Other drugs may be absorbed and chemically bound to the soft lens, thus decreasing the available dose of medication. With all types of contact lenses, drug contact with the eye is increased and more drug absorption may occur because of damage to the corneal epithelium caused by the lenses.

It is important to keep in mind that preservatives and the pH of a prescribed drug solution may cause dehydration or shape change in contact lenses, leading to discomfort and lens intolerance by the patient. In addition, eye drop suspensions may cause the build up of particulate matter, leading to discomfort, and ointments may change the relationship between the cornea and lens, leading to vision distortion.

Some eye drops, such as epinephrine, may actually discolor contact lenses, and some systemic drugs may affect contact lens wear. For example, rifampin, an antimicrobial drug, causes tears to become orange and stain the contact lens. To avoid these problems, you should explain to your patients who wear contacts that they should replace them with glasses for the duration of their treatment.

- Before putting any type of drop, ointment, or disc into the eye, wash your hands, put on sterile gloves, and explain the procedure to the patient and family. Most ointments are soothing to the eye, but some liquids or suspensions sting briefly. Be sure to warn patients of any possible discomfort they may experience to decrease anxiety.

- If the eye is crusty or needs cleaning, put on sterile gloves and use a cotton ball moistened in sterile, normal saline or another prescribed solution to gently clean the eyelid and lashes. Always wipe from the inner canthus to the outer canthus (i.e., from the nose to the side of the face) to prevent contaminating the other eye and the lacrimal (tear) duct.

To Administer Eye Drops:

- Give the patient a tissue.
- Have the patient sit or lie down and look up toward the ceiling.
- Carefully pull down the skin below the affected eye to expose the conjunctival sac.
- Administer the prescribed number of drops into the center of the conjunctival sac, being careful not to touch any eye structure. (To prevent blinking, approach the eye from below and outside the patient's visual field.)
- After applying the drops, have your patient close his or her eyes and press on the tear duct to prevent systemic absorption. The eyes should remain closed for about 1 minute to allow for distribution of the drug.

To Administer Eye Ointments:

- Apply ointment(s) at bedtime, if possible.
- Have the patient sit or lie down and look up.
- Expose the conjunctival sac and squeeze a ¼-inch strip of ointment into the sac.
- Have the patient close the eye for 2 to 3 minutes.
- Explain that it is normal for vision to be blurred for a few minutes after application.

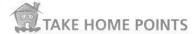

TAKE HOME POINTS

If a patient is to have an ointment instilled after an eye drop, wait 10 minutes before instilling the ointment to allow time for the drug contained in the drop to disperse.
Before squeezing out each dose of an ointment, warm the tube in your hand for a few minutes to make it flow more easily.
Contact lens wearers should substitute glasses for the duration of treatment with eye drops, ointments, or discs.

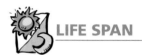

LIFE SPAN

The closed-eye technique may be used to administer eye drops to children. Have the child lie down and close his or her eyes. Place the drop on the inner canthus of the eyelid, and then have the child open the eye. Gravity will pull the drop into the eye.

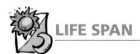

LIFE SPAN

The incidence of cataracts, retinal detachment, glaucoma, dry eyes, and other eye conditions increase with age. Older adults are also more likely to have cardiovascular disorders that may be aggravated by systemic absorption of eye drops or ointments. Anxiety and confusion is increased when eye conditions associated with blindness, such as glaucoma, are diagnosed. As a result, both written and oral instructions are necessary for patient education.

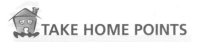

TAKE HOME POINTS

Brinzolamide (Azopt) 1% ophthalmic suspension is effective in treating primary open-angle glaucoma (POAG) and ocular hypertension (OH).

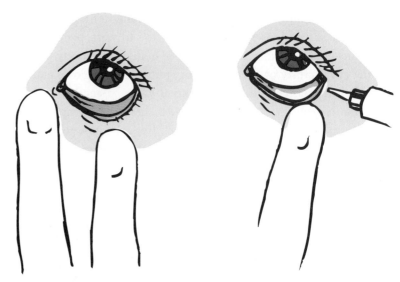

Eye ointment administration. *Redrawn from Kee JL, Hayes, ER:* Pharmacology: a nursing process approach, *ed 3, Philadelphia, 1997, WB Saunders.*

To Administer Medicated Discs:

• Remove any medicated discs already present in the eye. (To remove a disc, wear gloves, expose the conjunctival sac with one hand, and use your other thumb and forefinger to gently pinch the disc and lift it out of the eye.)

• Open the package carefully and press one fingertip against the disc so that it sticks to the finger.

• Position the disc carefully so that the convex (i.e., outward curve) side is on the fingertip.

• Ask the patient to look up and expose the conjunctival sac with your other hand.

• Place the disc into the sac so that it floats between the iris and lower eyelid.

• Pull the lower lid out and over the disc until it is covered. You should not be able to see the disc once it has been placed in the eye.

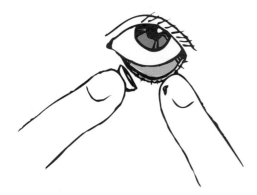

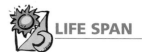

Families of older adults should be taught about the drugs being administered to their relatives and how to give them correctly. This is especially important if the older adult has arthritis, Parkinson's disease, or some other condition that may interfere with the ability to self-administer eye medications.

After applying eye drugs using any of these methods, gently wipe any excess drug off the eyelid, from inner to outer canthus. If an eye patch is prescribed, secure it without putting pressure on the eye. Then remove your gloves, dispose of any soiled equipment appropriately, and wash your hands. Next, document the dose and any visual changes or adverse effects. Finally, be sure to discuss the purpose of the drug, drug action, side effects, and administration techniques with the patient.

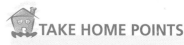
TAKE HOME POINTS

- Always wipe excess drugs from an eye from inner to outer canthus.
- Have the patient demonstrate self-administration of the next dose.

Do You UNDERSTAND?

DIRECTIONS: **Fill in the labeled boxes to complete each sentence: When administering eye drops or ointments, you should:**

Always

1. _____
2. _____
3. _____
4. _____

Never

5. _____
6. _____
7. _____
8. _____

Answers: 1. **Use the dropper provided;** 2. **Check the label for the words** *ophthalmic* or *optic;* 3. **Verify what abbreviations are acceptable in your institution;** 4. **Double check the meaning of abbreviations with the prescriber;** 5. **Place drops or ointments directly on the cornea;** 6. **Touch any part of the eye with droppers or tubes;** 7. **Dose the unaffected eye;** 8. **Let someone else use the medication.**

DIRECTIONS: **Unscramble the word in parentheses to fill in the blanks.**

9. *Optic* means _____. *(eey)*

10. *Otic* means _____. *(rae)*

11. Wait _____ minutes between drops of different drugs. *(vife)*

12. After an eye drop, wait _____ minutes before placing ointment in the same eye. *(net)*

13. Most eye drops have a _____ month shelf life. *(rehte)*

14. Use eye drops for only the _____ illness. *(tenurcr)*

15. Timolol plus systemic beta blockers may equal _____. *(daracbaryid)*

16. Discard the first _____ inch of ophthalmic ointment when opening a new tube. *(4/1)*

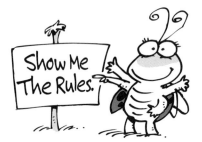

Show Me The Rules.

DIRECTIONS: **Fill in the blanks to complete the rules.**

17. RULE 1: Before administering eye drops, wash your _____ and put on _____.

18. RULE 2: Always wipe from the _____ to the outer canthus.

19. RULE 3: Always place eye medication in the _____ sac.

20. RULE 4: Afterwards, have the patient close the _____ for 1 minute.

21. RULE 5: To prevent systemic absorption, press on the _____ _____.

22. RULE 6: The best time to apply ointments is at _____.

DIRECTIONS: **These are the final answers. Complete the questions.**

23. Answer: Soft contact lens
    Question: What may absorb eye drops and create a sustained _____?

24. Answer: Glasses
    Question: What are substituted for contact lenses when _____?

25. Answer: Cardiovascular disease
    Question: What problems may be aggravated in the older adults by systemic absorption of _____?

What IS an Ear Medication?

An *ear medication* is used to relieve pain, treat external canal inflammation or infection, and soften cerumen (i.e., earwax) for removal. These drugs come in drop form and must be in direct contact with otic tissue to be effective.

What You NEED TO KNOW

When giving ear drops, be sure the container is labeled for *otic* or *auric* use only. Occasionally, abbreviations will be used to indicate which ear is to receive the dose: AS indicates the left ear, AD indicates the right ear, and AU indicates both ears. Use of these abbreviations is not as common as use of the abbreviations for eye medications. Therefore you should be familiar with the abbreviations used in your facility and always double check the meaning of the abbreviation with the prescribing health care provider.

The structures of the internal ear are very sensitive to temperature extremes. Sudden changes of temperature within the ear or near the tympanic membrane (ear drum) may cause extreme dizziness, nausea, or ataxia (i.e., a staggering gait). To prevent the development of these conditions, you should warm ear drops to body temperature before administering them. Because drugs given into the ear are topical, drug-to-drug interactions are rare. However, benzocaine drops (anesthetic) inhibit the action of otic sulfa drugs, so these medications should not be given together.

TAKE HOME POINTS

- Warm ear drops to body temperature by placing them in a pocket for a few minutes or by running warm water over the bottom of the container. If warm water is used, do not allow the water to reach the upper part of the container to prevent contaminating the contents.
- Do not use topical preparations for ears when there is a known rupture of the eardrum.
- Maintain sterility of drug preparations given into the ear. Although the external ear is not sterile, the eardrum may be ruptured and introduction of a contaminated solution could cause a middle ear infection.
- Ear drops are more easily given by someone other than the patient.

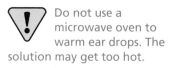 Do not use a microwave oven to warm ear drops. The solution may get too hot.

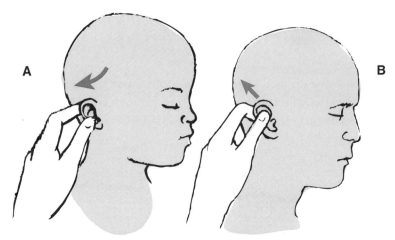

A, On a child, straighten the external ear canal by pulling down and back on the pinna of the ear. **B,** On an adult, straighten it by pulling up and back on the pinna of the ear.

What You DO

- To decrease anxiety, you should explain the procedure to the patient and the family before administering ear drops. (Tell them that the drops will be warmed to body temperature and why.)
- Place the patient in a sitting position, with the head tilted slightly toward the unaffected side, or have the patient lie on his or her side with the affected ear up. (Be sure the patient is comfortable.)
- Inspect the ear canal. If there is impacted ear wax, it must be removed before use of antibacterial ear drops so that the drops have good contact with the skin of the external canal.

To Administer Ear Drops:

- Expose the ear canal and instill the prescribed number of drops, taking care not to contaminate the dropper.
- Temporarily place a cotton ball over the ear canal to prevent the drops from leaking out of the ear.
- Instruct the patient to remain in the same position for 2 to 3 minutes to allow time for the drug to flow into the ear canal.

If the external ear canal is obstructed with edema, a gauze ear wick can be inserted past the swollen segment of the canal and the drops applied to the outside part of the gauze wick. The drug is absorbed along the path of the wick into the depths of the canal. When the edema subsides (usually in about 48 hours), the wick can be removed and drops applied directly into the canal using the procedure previously described. An ear wick may require an additional prescription.

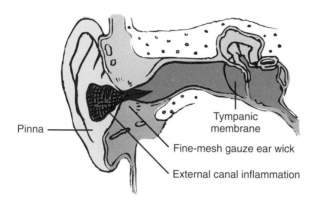

Pinna

Tympanic membrane

Fine-mesh gauze ear wick

External canal inflammation

LIFE SPAN

If the patient is over the age of 3 years, gently grasp the pinna (i.e., upper outer external ear) and pull up and back to see ear canal and make sure the drops reach the affected area. For a child under 3 years old, pull down and back on the pinna to straighten the ear canal and allow the drops to reach the affected area.

⚠ Never obstruct the ear canal with a dropper or force any solution into the ear. To do so may damage the tympanic membrane.

Do You UNDERSTAND?

DIRECTIONS: Circle the phrase below each statement that completes it correctly.

1. To be effective, ear drops must be _____ otic tissue.
   a. in direct contact with   b. warmed to increase blood flow to
2. The correct abbreviation for the right ear is _____.
   a. AS   b. AU   c. AD
3. Sudden changes in temperature of ear structures may cause _____
   _____.
   a. shivering and vomiting   b. dizziness and ataxia
4. Ear drops should always be warmed to _____.
   a. body temperature   b. room temperature
5. Warm ear drops by _____.
   a. using body heat   b. using the microwave
6. To instill ear drops, pull the pinna of the ear _____ in an adult.
   a. up and back   b. down and back   c. forward and down

TAKE HOME POINTS

- Pull up and back on the pinna for an older child or adult and down and back for a child under 3 years of age.
- If there is a discharge from the ear, do not place drops into an external ear canal without checking with the prescribing health care provider. The eardrum may be ruptured, and the fluid may be CSF. Check the drainage for glucose and notify the provider.
- After using antibacterial or drying ear drops, you may dry the ear canal for 30 seconds with a hair dryer set on cool or low heat. Hold the dryer at least 24 inches from the ear.
- Instruct patients not to share ear drops with others to prevent cross contamination.

Answers: 1. a; 2. c; 3. b; 4. a; 5. a; 6. a.

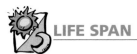

LIFE SPAN

Saline sprays or drops are a safer decongestant alternative for children and older adults than many OTC nasal drops or sprays containing sympathomimetics. Older patients may actually become addicted to sympathomimetics, because these drugs produce effects resembling those resulting from stimulation of the sympathetic nervous system.

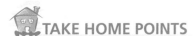

TAKE HOME POINTS

Decongestant drops and sprays used for more than 3 days cause a rebound effect in which nasal congestion increases.

TAKE HOME POINTS

Azelastine (Astelin) nasal spray is effective for treating seasonal allergic rhinitis.
Nasal mupirocin is effective treatment for *Staphylococcus aureus*.

What ARE Nose Drops and Sprays?

Nose drops and sprays are used to shrink swollen mucous membranes, loosen secretions, moisten nasal passages, or to treat nasal or sinus infections. In addition, nose sprays are used as decongestants.

What You NEED TO KNOW

There are many over-the-counter (OTC) nasal decongestants available. Most contain sympathomimetics, medications that mimic the effects of sympathetic nervous system stimulation. If more than the recommended number of drops or sprays is used and excess decongestant solution is swallowed, serious systemic effects, such as tachycardia and palpitations, may develop.

What You DO

To Administer Nose Drops:

- Have the patient clear the nasal passages by blowing the nose gently, unless contraindicated by increased intracranial pressure.
- Place the patient in the supine position, with the head tilted back and a small pillow under the shoulders. To ensure flow to the frontal and maxillary sinuses, have the patient turn his or her head toward the affected side.
- Wash your hands and put on gloves.
- With your nondominant hand, push upward on the end of the patient's nose to open the nostrils.
- Instill the drops just inside the nostril on the affected side (without touching it).
- Discard any remaining drug in the dropper before returning the dropper to the container.
- Have the patient remain in position for 3 to 5 minutes to ensure distribution of the drug.
- Provide a tissue to assist with removal of any drug that pools in the throat or mouth.

To Administer Nose Sprays:

- Have the patient sit upright and tilt his or her head back slightly.
- Follow instructions on the label. Instructions may include directing the patient to close one nostril, tilt his or her head to the affected side, inhale through the affected side after spraying, or hold the breath for several seconds after using the spray.
- If possible, the patient should self-administer the spray to control the amount and coordinate inhalation as it enters the nasal passages.

Do You UNDERSTAND?

DIRECTIONS: Here are the results. List the most likely cause.

1. Result: Rebound nasal congestion

   Cause: _____

2. Result: Tachycardia and palpitations

   Cause: _____

3. Result: Yellow or green nasal discharge

   Cause: _____

4. Result: Contaminated nasal spray

   Cause a: _____

   Cause b: _____

   Cause c: _____

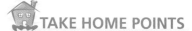

TAKE HOME POINTS

- Inform adults, especially older patients, that decongestant drops and sprays used for more than 3 days can cause a rebound effect in which nasal congestion increases.
- Warn patients that to avoid spreading infection they should never use another person's nose drops or nasal sprays.
- Use OTC nose drops or nasal sprays for only one illness, because it is easy for these medications to become contaminated with bacteria.
- Tell your patients that a change in color or consistency of mucous discharge can indicate a worsening problem. (Yellow or green nasal discharge indicates an infection.)

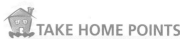

TAKE HOME POINTS

Nicotine nasal sprays are most effective in helping people to stop smoking if the person is obese, a member of a minority group, or highly dependent on smoking.

Answers: 1. Use of nasal decongestant drops or spray for more than 3 days; 2. Using excess decongestant drops or sprays and swallowing them; 3. Infection; 4. a. Touching the nostril with the dropper; b. Using the drops/spray for more than one illness episode; c. Not discarding remaining drug in the dropper before returning it to the container.

References

Alper BS: Evidence-based medicine. Choosing an antibiotic for otitis externa, *Clin Advisor* 7(3):126, 2004.

Berger WE, White MV: Efficacy of azelastine nasal spray in patients with unsatisfactory response to loratadine, *Ann Allergy Asthma Immunol* 91(2):205-11, 2003.

Cvetkovic RS, Pery CM: Brinzolamide: a review of its use in the management of primary open-angle glaucoma and ocular hypertension, *Drugs Aging* 20(12): 919-47, 2003.

Lally RT, Lanz E, Schrock CG: Rapid control of an outbreak of *Staphylococcus aureus* on a neonatal intensive care department using standard infection control practices and nasal mupirocin, *Am J Infect Control* 3(91):44-7, 2004.

Lerman C, Kaufmann V, Rukstalis M et al: Individualizing nicotine replacement therapy for the treatment of tobacco dependence: a randomized trial, *Ann Intern Med* 140(6):426-33, I-47, 2004.

NCLEX® Review

Circle the correct answer.

1. You have been asked to administer timolol 0.25%
   1 gtt, bid, OU, to a patient with glaucoma. You
   place one drop in:
   1 Both eyes
   2 Left eye
   3 Right eye
   4 Both ears

2. You instruct a patient how to self-administer
   eye drops that were prescribed to treat his ocular
   infection. You know the patient understands how
   to do this correctly when he says:
   1 "If my wife catches this infection, I'll let her use
   my drops."
   2 "I won't touch any part of my eye when I put in
   the drops."
   3 "I'll hold my eye open with my fingers and let
   the drop fall on my eyeball."
   4 "I'll wipe my eyes from the side of my face to
   the nose each time."

3. Mr. Carter is to receive two different eye drops
   each evening. You advise his wife to:
   1 "Give the first drop, wait a minute, then give the
   next one."
   2 "Give the first drop, wait until it stops stinging,
   and give the next one."
   3 "Give both drops at the same time."
   4 "Give one, then wait 5 minutes and give the
   other."

4. When instructing Mrs. Potter, a patient who is
   prescribed timolol eye gel, 0.5% qd, you advise her
   to instill ¼ inch of the gel:
   1 After breakfast
   2 Upon waking in the morning

   3 At bedtime
   4 After supper

5. Sally Charles, a wearer of contact lenses, has
   developed "pink eye," a bacterial infection of
   the eye. The physician has prescribed antibiotic
   drops bid. Sally asks you if she should continue
   to wear her contacts, and you correctly respond
   that:
   1 She should continue to wear her contact lenses
   to get maximum effect from the drug.
   2 She should not wear her contact lenses until
   after she had had three doses of eye drops.
   3 She may wear her lenses if her eyes are not
   painful.
   4 She may not wear her contact lenses for the
   duration of time she is receiving eye drops.

6. You are teaching Mrs. Finny how to give ear drops
   to her 2-year-old child. You know the teaching has
   been effective if Mrs. Finny states that she will:
   1 Tilt the child's head back to give the drops.
   2 Pull the pinna of the ear down and back to
   straighten the external canal.
   3 Pull the pinna of the ear up and back to
   straighten the external canal.
   4 Turn the head toward the affected side and give
   the drops after pulling the earlobe down.

7. To warm ear drops, you may:
   1 Hold them in your hands or carry them in your
   pocket until they warm to body temperature.
   2 Warm them to room temperature by allowing
   them to remain on the drug cart at all times.
   3 Heat them to body temperature in the
   microwave oven.
   4 Hold them under hot, running water until the
   container is hot to the touch.

8. As you are preparing to administer antibiotic ear drops to Mr. Garrison, you observe a new, blood-tinged discharge from his left ear. You should:
   1 Administer the drops and chart your findings.
   2 Hold the drops until the physician is notified.
   3 Irrigate the ear to remove the discharge, then give the drops.
   4 Place a wick in the ear canal and administer the drops on the wick.

9. To ensure flow to the frontal and maxillary sinuses when giving nose drops, you should position the patient in the supine position, with the head tilted back and a small pillow under the shoulders. You should also ask the patient to:
   1 Turn the head toward the affected side.
   2 Hold the head in a neutral position.
   3 Keep the neck flexed.
   4 Turn the head toward the unaffected side.

10. To prevent contaminating nose drops, you should:
    1 Open the nostrils by pushing on the end of the nose on the affected side.
    2 Place the drops just inside the nostril on the affected side, without touching it.
    3 Provide a clean tissue for the patient to sneeze into to prevent spreading droplets.
    4 Have the patient remain in position for 3 to 5 minutes after giving the drops.

11. True or False? Medications prescribed for use in the eye are known as "otic" medications.

12. Fill in the blank. Administration of eye drops includes pulling down the skin below the affected eye to expose the _____ sac.

13. Short answer: If drainage from the ear is positive for glucose, where might this drainage be coming from? _____

14. Short answer: Decongestant drops and sprays can cause rebound effect. What is the usual maximum number of days when rebound effect will begin to occur? _____

15. Fill in the blank: Many over-the-counter (OTC) medications that are nasal decongestants contain sympathomimetics, which can cause the heart rate to _____.

NCLEX® Review Answers

1. **1** OU is the abbreviation for both eyes. The abbreviation for the left eye is OS. The abbreviation for the right eye is OD. The abbreviations for the ears are AS, AD, and AU.

2. **2** Not touching the eye prevents contamination of the drops. Eye drops should never be shared to prevent cross contamination or possible injury. Give drops into the conjunctival sac, not on the eyeball, to prevent pain. To prevent cross contamination, wipe from the nose (inner canthus) to the side of the face (outer canthus).

3. **4** Giving the drugs 5 minutes apart allows time for each drug to be effective. More than 1 minute's time is necessary to prevent diluting or washing away the first drop and giving both drugs at the same time would wash away or dilute the drugs. Not all eye drops cause discomfort.

4. **3** Gels or ointments may interfere with vision temporarily, so it is safer to use them at bedtime.

5. **4** Discontinuing wearing contact lenses for the duration of treatment enhances the effectiveness of treatment, prevents reinfection, and decreases discomfort. Wearing contacts will likely cause more discomfort and may decrease the effectiveness of treatment. Wearing contacts may also cause reinfection.

6. **2** Pulling the pinna down and back will allow the drops to flow into the external canal. Tilting the child's head back does not allow the mother to see the ear canal, and pulling the pinna up and back is the procedure for an adult or child over the age of 3 years. The affected ear will be facing away from, not toward, the mother if the head is turned to the affected side.

7. **1** Warming drops in your hands or pocket prevents the dizziness, nausea, and vomiting that could result from using cold drops. Drops need to be at body temperature. Never heat drops in the microwave—they may get too hot. Use warm water (not hot) across the bottom of the container; the container should never feel more than lukewarm. Drops may need to be refrigerated between administrations.

8. **2** Hold the drops. Test the fluid for glucose (indicating the presence of cerebrospinal fluid [CSF]), and notify the physician of the results. You would not give the drops because Mr. Garrison may have a ruptured eardrum or CSF leak. If the eardrum is ruptured, irrigation could do further damage. A wick is used with a blocked external canal and may require a physician's prescription.

9. **1** Turning the head to the affected side allows the drops to enter the sinuses. Holding the head in a neutral position would cause the drops to flow down the throat. If the neck is flexed, the drops will flow out of the nose. If you turn the head toward the unaffected side, the drops would enter the wrong sinuses.

10. **2** Avoiding touching the dropper to anything will prevent contamination of the drops. Pushing on the affected side would not prevent contamination. Sneezing will not contaminate the drops; the dropper is returned immediately to the container after instilling the drops. Having the patient remain in position 3 to 5 minutes allows the drops to flow into the proper area, but it does not prevent contamination.

11. False. Otic medications are for the ear.

12. conjunctival.

13. cerebrospinal fluid.

14. after 3 days.

15. increase or become tachycardic.

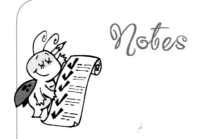

Notes

11  Administration of Rectal and Vaginal Medications

What You WILL LEARN

After reading this chapter, you will know how to do the following:

✔ Identify rectal and vaginal medications.
✔ Calculate prescribed amounts of rectal and vaginal medications based on availability and prescription.

What IS a Rectal Medication?

Rectal medications are inserted into the rectum in the form of suppositories and enemas. Suppositories are easily melted preparations in a firm base. They have front ends that are tapered or rounded to facilitate insertion, and smaller sizes are available for administration to infants and children. Liquid medications may be given by enema and are designed to be retained and absorbed by the rectal mucosa for a given amount of time.

What You NEED TO KNOW

Rectal Suppositories

The rectal route of drug administration is used to achieve both local and systemic effects. For example, rectal suppositories may be administered to:

• Promote a bowel movement (local effect)
• Reduce temperature (systemic effect)

- Treat nausea (systemic effect)
- Control pain (systemic effects)

Rectal medications are extremely useful when your patients cannot tolerate oral medications or fluids. However, the rectal method of medication administration is among those least preferred by patients because they fear discomfort and embarrassment. In reality, properly administered rectal medications will cause minimal discomfort for your patients, and you can reduce their embarrassment by encouraging self-administration of the medication.

Enemas

Most medicated enemas are packaged in ready-to-administer sets and accompanied by administration instructions. Oil retention and Kayexalate are examples of the kind of medicated enemas that you will administer to your patients.

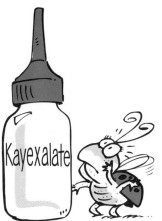

What You DO

To Administer Rectal Suppositories

- Review the prescription and check your patient's record for information concerning allergies, rectal bleeding, or recent surgery.
- Gather clean gloves, linen protectors, tissues, suppository, water-soluble lubricant, and the patient's medication record.
- If necessary, put on protective devices (e.g., gown, mask and goggles).
- Wash your hands, check the patient's identification (ID bracelet), and ask that the patient to void before insertion.

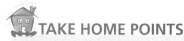

CULTURE

When administering rectal medications, you must be aware of certain cultural-sensitivity issues. Remember that a patient's willingness to participate in a procedure or accept a medication may•be a reflection of his or her cultural values.

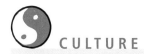

TAKE HOME POINTS

Advantages of rectal medication administration:
1. Prevents upper gastrointestinal irritation.
2. Medications are well absorbed across mucosal surface of rectum.
3. Excellent bloodstream levels (titers) of medication obtained.

CULTURE

Be aware of certain cultural sensitivity issues, such as your patient's level of personal modesty and his or her perception of what constitutes improper touching or a violation of personal space. A patient's willingness to participate in a procedure or accept a medication may be a reflection of cultural values.

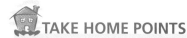

TAKE HOME POINTS

To prevent melting, store suppositories in a refrigerator until just before administration.

- Explain the procedure, including special points about retention.
- Provide privacy and drape the patient, with only the anal area exposed.
- Help the patient to lie on his or her side. (Based on the anatomy of the sigmoid colon, the left side is recommended.)
- If condition permits, have the patient bring his or her knees up to the chest (for maximum administration).
- Apply your gloves, examine the condition of the anus, and palpate rectal walls as necessary.
- If you detect fecal impaction, follow agency policy for removal. (If it is necessary to remove an impaction, change your gloves and wash your hands after the procedure.)
- Instruct the patient to take slow deep breaths to help relax the anal sphincter.
- Separate the buttocks and gently insert the suppository, lubricated with water-soluble lubricant, past the internal anal sphincter (about 4 inches in adults and 2 inches in children) and against rectal wall.
- Withdraw your finger and wipe the anal area with a tissue.
- Discard your gloves and wash your hands.
- Instruct the patient to remain on his or her side for 5 minutes.
- Place a call light and a bedpan or bedside commode within the patient's reach.
- Repeat the procedure if suppository is expelled.
- Document the medication administration on the patient's medication record.
- Observe for effects of the suppository (e.g., bowel movement, fever reduction, relief of nausea) in 30 minutes or within a specified time following insertion.
- Document the effects and how well the procedure was tolerated.

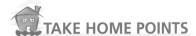

TAKE HOME POINTS

Antimigraine medication sumatriptan (Imitrex), given in a 25-mg suppository form, is a useful alternative route for some patients.

When using a glove, turn the glove inside out after withdrawal from the rectum. This prevents the spread of microorganisms.

Insert lubricated suppository past the anal sphincter. Repeat procedure if suppository is expelled. Assess for drug effects after insertion.

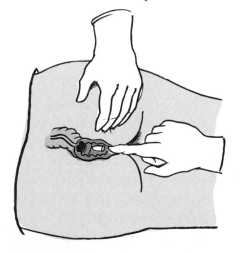

Age-Specific Considerations

There are several considerations when administering rectal suppositories to certain age groups:

Infants and children. Because of lack of control of the anal sphincter, infants and some older children may not be able to retain a rectal suppository. Therefore you may have to stay with younger patients and gently hold their buttocks together until the medication takes effect. Children are often frightened by invasive procedures and may resist administration of the suppository. If this is the case, reassure the child and, if necessary, have his or her parent assist you in the procedure.

Older adults. Your older patients may also have decreased sphincter control and an inability to retain a suppository. If a suppository cannot be retained after a second attempt, notify the prescribing professional so that the drug may be given by another route, if possible.

To Administer Enemas

- Gather clean gloves; linen protectors; tissues; prepackaged, disposable enema; water-soluble lubricant; and the patient's medication record.
- If necessary, put on protective devices (e.g., gown, mask, and goggles).
- Wash your hands, check the patient's ID and ask the patient to void before inserting.
- Explain the procedure, including special points about retention.
- Provide privacy and drape the patient, with only the anal area exposed.
- Help the patient to lie on either side and drape, with only the anal area exposed.
- Apply linen-saver to bedding (in case of leakage).
- Apply your gloves, examine the condition of the anus, and palpate rectal walls as necessary.
- If you detect fecal impaction, follow agency policy for removal. (If it is necessary to remove an impaction, change your gloves and wash your hands after the procedure.)
- Instruct the patient to take slow deep breaths to help relax the anal sphincter.
- Separate the buttocks, and gently insert the prelubricated enema tip past the internal sphincter (3 to 4 inches in adults and 1 to 3 inches in pediatric patients).
- Squeeze the bottle until the solution has entered the rectum (a small amount of fluid will remain in the bottle).
- Reinforce the necessity for retention.
- Document the procedure, including how the patient tolerated it.

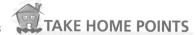

TAKE HOME POINTS

Because medications administered by enema are meant to be retained by the patient, they will be small in amount.

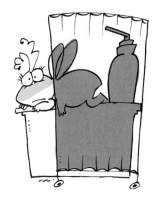

Age-Specific Considerations

There are considerations when administering enemas to certain age groups:

Infants and children. Because of lack of control of anal sphincter, this is not an appropriate route for delivering medications to infants. Although enemas are appropriate for older children, they may also be unable to retain the solution or refuse to allow you to administer it. As in the case of rectal suppository administration, reassure the child and have his or her parent assist you in the procedure, if necessary.

Older adults. Your older patients may be unable to retain the solution because of decreased sphincter control. If this is the case, notify the prescribing professional so that the drug may be given by another route, if possible.

Do You UNDERSTAND?

DIRECTIONS : **Select the best answer.**

1. A rectal suppository administered to a 4-year-old child should be inserted:
   a. About 4 inches
   b. About 2 inches
   c. As far as it will go
   d. Until the child resists
2. If a suppository is expelled *twice*, you should:
   a. Repeat the procedure.
   b. Tell patients that they *must not* expel it again.
   c. Record in your notes that the suppository could not be retained.
   d. Notify the prescribing professional to see if the drug can be administered by another route.

DIRECTIONS: **Unscramble the following sentences.**

3. Tapstein solhud eb doefrfe teh toprpotuniy ot fels-tiamdnrise semnea fi yeht ear yplachsily leab ot od os.
4. Telrca rispuoypsoies yam eb sardeteminid ot meproot a owleb veetmomn, cedrue rateempetur, retat asunea, nad rotlnco inap.
5. Dhelcdrin rea netfo gedntfrihe yb inavvsie ropdercues; riovdep asresneurac.

TAKE HOME POINTS

- When administering rectal medications, consider the patient's age in regard to his or her ability to retain the drug for the required time.
- If condition permits, allow the patient to self-administer the medication.
- Observe the patient after administration for 30 minutes, and record the effects of the procedure.
- If the patient is unable to retain the drug, notify the prescribing professional to see if the drug may be administered by another route.

Answers: **1. b; 2. d; 3. Patients should be offered the opportunity to self-administer enemas if they are physically able to do so; 4. Rectal suppositories may be administered to promote a bowel movement, reduce temperature, treat nausea, and control pain; 5. Children are often frightened by invasive procedures; provide reassurance.**

What IS a Vaginal Medication?

Vaginal medications are inserted into the vaginal canal in the form of suppositories, jellies, creams, or foams. Administration at bedtime will help prevent gravity drainage. They are used for contraceptive purposes and to treat infections. Although most of your patients will prefer to self-administer these medications, you should be familiar with all administration procedures.

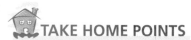
TAKE HOME POINTS

Five-day treatment with intravaginal metronidazole is effective for bacterial vaginosis during pregnancy.

What You NEED TO KNOW

When administering vaginal medications, you should review the prescribing professional's order and check the patient's medical record for allergies. Remember to check whether the patient has recently given birth or undergone vaginal surgery.

What You DO

To Administer Vaginal Suppositories

- Gather clean gloves, tissues, suppository, water-soluble lubricant, perianal pad, and the patient's medication record.
- Wash your hands, check the patient's ID, and explain the procedure.
- Have the patient void before insertion.
- Provide privacy and help the patient to lie on her back with knees flexed.
- Place a pillow under the patient's hips.
- Drape to maintain privacy.
- Apply gloves.
- Use a lamp or flashlight to see the vaginal opening clearly.
- Spread labia and cleanse with cotton balls and warm water, using single downward strokes.
- Gently insert the lubricated suppository.
- Provide a clean perianal pad to absorb any drainage.
- Have the patient remain in a supine position for 5 to 10 minutes following insertion (to maximize absorption).
- Document the procedure on the patient's medication record.

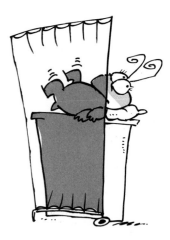

To Administer Creams, Jellies, and Foams

- Fill the applicator according to the manufacturer's instructions (if the medication does not come with a prefilled applicator).
- Gather clean gloves, tissues, suppository, water-soluble lubricant, perianal pad, and the patient's medication record.
- Wash your hands, check the patient's ID, and explain the procedure.
- Have the patient void before insertion.
- Provide privacy and assist the patient to lie on her back with knees flexed.
- Place a pillow under the patient's hips.
- Drape to maintain privacy.
- Apply gloves.
- Use a lamp or flashlight to see the vaginal opening clearly.
- Spread labia and cleanse with cotton balls and warm water, using single downward strokes.
- Gently insert the lubricated applicator, aiming it down and back along the full length of the vagina.
- Push the plunger to its full length, and gently remove the applicator (with the plunger depressed).
- Provide a clean perianal pad to absorb any drainage.
- Have the patient remain in a supine position for 5 to 10 minutes following insertion.
- Document the procedure on the patient's medication record.

LIFE SPAN

When working with children, you should have a parent or support person available to assist in the procedure.

When working with older patients, remember that they may be unable to self-administer the medication and therefore may require assistance.

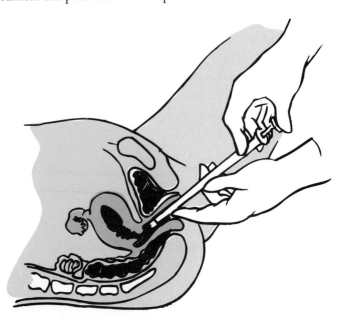

Do You UNDERSTAND?

DIRECTIONS: **Select the best answer.**

1. The reason that the patient should remain supine after administration of vaginal medications is because:
   a. The vagina lacks sphincter control, and medications will drain out.
   b. The patient will not experience cramping in this position.
   c. If the patient tries to get up, the medication may make her dizzy.
   d. The reason is unknown.

DIRECTIONS: **Fill in the blanks.**

2. Gently insert _____ _____, aiming it down and back along the full length of the vagina.
3. Administration at _____ will help prevent gravity drainage of vaginal suppositories.
4. Be sure to note whether the patient who is to receive vaginal medication has recently given _____ or has undergone _____ _____.
5. Use a _____ or _____ to see the vaginal opening clearly.

References

Desai DH, Shirley KL, Penzak SR: Pharmacokinetics in healthy volunteers of sumatriptan 25-mg oral treatment versus 25-mg extemporaneous suppository. *Int J Pharm Compound* 7(6):481-4, 2003.

Elsley K, Chan LC, Waldrop JB: Advisor forum: fighting vaginal infections, *Clin Advisor* 7(3):80, 85, 2004.

Yudin MH, Landers DV, Meyn L et al: Clinical and cervical Cytokine response to treatment with oral or vaginal metronidazole for bacterial vaginosis during pregnancy: a randomized trial, *Obstet Gynecol* 102(3):527-34, 2003.

Answers: 1. a; 2. lubricated applicator; 3. bedtime; 4. birth, vaginal surgery; 5. lamp, flashlight.

Notes

NCLEX® Review

Circle the correct answer.

1. The purpose of a rectal suppository can be to:
   1 Promote defecation
   2 Relieve nausea
   3 Neither 1 nor 2
   4 Both 1 and 2

2. Rectal suppositories may not be retained by older adults because:
   1 The rectum in older adults is too small to accommodate suppositories.
   2 Many older adults experience loss of sphincter control.
   3 Older adults resent this intrusion on their privacy.
   4 They react to the pain of insertion.

3. Liquid medications administered rectally by enema:
   1 Are meant to be expelled
   2 Are given only when there is no other available route
   3 Are meant to be retained and absorbed
   4 Have very little therapeutic effect

4. In most cases, vaginal medications are most effective if they are:
   1 Self-administered
   2 Administered in the early morning
   3 Administered with patient seated on the toilet
   4 Administered at bedtime

5. The reason a deep plunger is used when administering vaginal medication is because:
   1 The plunger ensures placement of medication deep in the vagina.
   2 It is more comfortable.
   3 It ensures fewer side effects.
   4 Cramping is less likely.

6. Short answer: Why are the tips of suppositories tapered or round? _____

7. Short answer: Is a rectal suppository of acetaminophen (Tylenol) given for its local or systemic effects to a patient who has a fever? _____

8. Fill in the blank: Based on the anatomy of the sigmoid colon, a rectal suppository should be administered with the patient lying on his or her _____ side.

9. True or False? Vaginal medications are best administered and absorbed with the female in the upright and standing position. _____

10. True or False? In an adult, you should insert the enema tip 6 to 9 inches past the internal sphincter. _____

NCLEX® Review Answers

1. **4** The purpose of a rectal suppository can be to promote defecation *and* relieve nausea.

2. **2** Many older adults experience loss of sphincter control and cannot retain suppositories. An older adult's rectum is *not* too small for suppositories. Older adults may resent the intrusion on their privacy, but this is unlikely to affect the physical ability to retain a suppository. Insertion is not usually painful unless the patient has hemorrhoids; if there are hemorrhoids, they are more likely to *retain* a suppository as a reaction to pain.

3. **3** The medication should be retained and absorbed, not expelled. Liquid medications administered by

enema may be given when other routes are available, but the rectal route may be preferred for various reasons. These medications have a therapeutic effect when correctly administered.

4. **4** Administering vaginal medications at bedtime prevents loss of the medication through excessive movement or an upright position and makes the medications more effective. Self-administration may be less effective if the patient has poor motor skills or fails to learn the correct technique of insertion.

5. **1** A deep plunger is used when administering vaginal medication because it ensures placement of medication deep in the vagina. A deeper plunger is momentarily more uncomfortable. The depth of the plunger will not ensure fewer side effects. Cramping does not usually occur with vaginal medications.

6. To ease insertion so you do not need to waste medications.

7. Systemic effects.

8. left.

9. False. Lie on the back with knees flexed to prevent gravity drainage.

10. False. 3 to 4 inches for an adult.

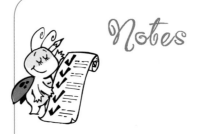

Notes

Intravenous Therapy

What You WILL LEARN

After reading this chapter, you will know how to do the following:

✔ Identify common intravenous fluids and principles of flow.
✔ Recognize differences between modes of administration, such as piggyback, push, and titration.
✔ Calculate intravenous rates based on patient prescription and drop factor.

This chapter discusses intravenous (IV) fluids, insertion procedure, calculating IV infusion rate, titration of IV fluids, IV piggyback, and IV push.

What IS an Intravenous Fluid?

An *IV fluid* is administered into the circulatory system through a vein. The IV route is the preferred route for fluid and electrolyte maintenance and/or replacement and medication administration (particularly antibiotics and pain medications). Medications are rapidly absorbed from this route, and the need for repeated intramuscular (IM) injections is eliminated. Although solutions and/or medications must be prescribed by a physician or an advanced practical nurse, the administration and regulation of IV fluids and/or medications and the maintenance of the IV catheter and dressing are the clinical nurse's responsibility. When continuous IV fluids are not necessary, a lock device (often called a *heparin lock* or *saline lock* or *INT*) may be used. These lock devices (the catheter and a cap) provide greater patient mobility.

What You NEED TO KNOW

IV solutions may be prescribed for a variety of reasons, including fluid replacement and maintenance of electrolyte balance. Fluid replacement is necessary when the patient is not able to meet oral intake requirements, such as is seen with vomiting, diarrhea, hemorrhaging, nasogastric suction, postoperative recovery, chronic obstructive pulmonary disease, or burns.

Large volume IV solutions are packaged in glass containers or plastic bags (most common) with a 500 mL to 1000 mL capacity. Small volume bags (e.g., 50 mL, 100 mL, and 250 mL) are used to administer IV medications. An IV administration set is attached to the IV solution bag (this equipment varies, based on the infusion requirement) and to the IV catheter inserted in the patient to permit fluid to infuse into the patient. IV medications are administered by IV push, intermittently or continuously. Intermittent infusions can be administered alone or piggybacked onto a continuous infusion administration set. Different administration sets are required for glass containers (vented) versus bags (nonvented), intermittent versus continuous infusions that require piggyback medications, piggybacks (also referred to as secondary), specialty requirements (blood administration, low absorption, pump specific), and meter chambered (buretrol).

Parts of a Peripheral Catheter

Peripheral vascular access is commonly accomplished by inserting an over-the-needle catheter into a small peripheral vein found on the hand or forearm.

The catheter is hollow with a stylet (needle) threaded through the catheter, ending with a sharp tip that extends beyond the catheter edge. The stylet's sharp tip allows the skin and vein to be punctured while the stylet shaft adds rigidity to the catheter for ease of advancement into the vein. The catheter has a colored hub. The color identifies the catheter gauge. The flashback chamber permits the inserter to view blood when

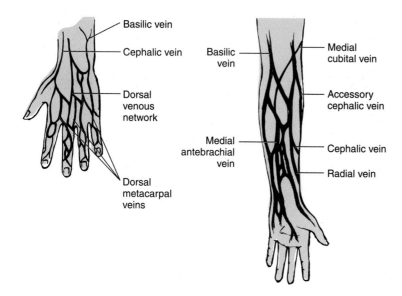

the vein is accessed. The air vent permits blood to flow into the flashback chamber. The Centers for Disease Control and Prevention (CDC) quidelines recommend 96-hour dwell time.

Another type of peripheral catheter is the butterfly. This is a stainless steel needle with soft pliable wings and an attached short extension tube. A butterfly is commonly used for blood draws, and single dose IV push medications.

Over-the-Needle Catheter

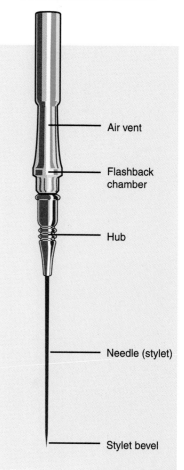

BUTTERFLY SET

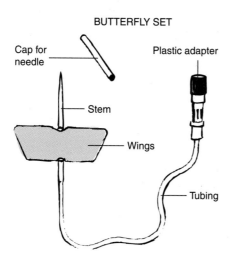

Central Venous Access

Central venous access requires a longer catheter inserted into a larger vein with the catheter tip located in a central vein (superior vena cava).

Central venous access devices are divided into three different types depending on length of use. *Short-term catheters,* such as the common subclavian multilumen or a pulmonary artery (Swan-Ganz), are commonly in place for less than 1 month. *Intermediate catheters,* such as a peripherally inserted central catheter (PICC) or a Hohn, are placed for 6 weeks or less. *Long-term catheters,* such as an implanted port or tunneled catheter (Hickman), can be left in place for longer than 6 weeks and possibly a year or more.

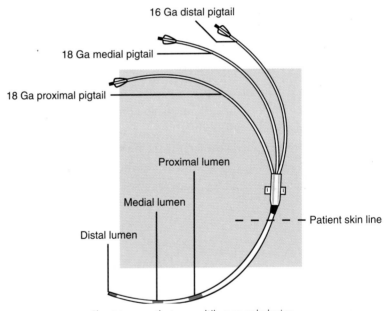

Short-term catheter: multilumen subclavian.

Hickman® and Leonard® Dual Lumen Catheters
(not drawn to scale)

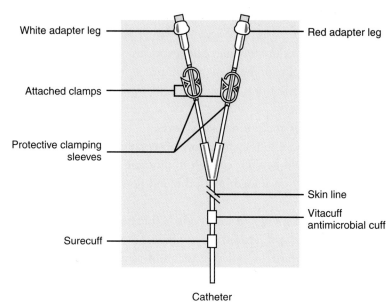

Long-term catheters: Hickman® and Leonard® dual lumen catheters.

PasV™ Port
Proximal Valve

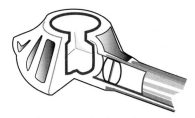

Long-term implanted port.

What You DO

Peripheral IV Catheter Insertion

- Confirm the patient's prescription for the solution type, volume, rate of flow.
- Collect the IV solution, appropriate administration set, two IV catheters (appropriate for administration requirements), IV start kit or skin prep solutions (alcohol wipes, Betadine solution or combination solution), tourniquet, moisture proof barrier, tape, and site dressing.

The Occupational Safety and Health Administration (OSHA) guidelines require the use of needle-protector systems and needle-free access systems.

The tourniquet should not be left in place longer than 2 minutes or the vein will become flat.

If your patient is allergic to iodine or shellfish, do not use Betadine.

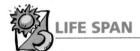 **LIFE SPAN**

In the elderly patient, apply tourniquet loosely over clothing to prevent overextention of the vein and to protect the skin from tearing or bruising. The prominent, large, firm vein in the elderly may be a poor choice because of poor ability to stabilize and increased resistance to puncture.

- Check the fluid for clarity and expiration date.
- Connect the IV tubing to the solution container, open roller clamp, and fill the tubing with solution (prime). Close roller clamp once the tubing is primed.
- Explain the procedure to your patient and his or her family members. Include the purpose of the therapy, duration of the therapy, the type of therapy, any restrictions to activity, and signs and symptoms that should be reported.
- Wash your hands and put on clean gloves.
- Apply tourniquet 4 to 6 inches above potential insertion location. The tourniquet should be tight enough to promote venous distention but not tight enough to impede arterial blood flow (radial pulse must be present).
- Select a soft- and springy-to-touch vein. Avoid bifurcations, valves, bony prominences, areas of flexion, arms with loss of motor or sensory function, arms with arteriovenous fistula, and arms affected by CVA or mastectomy. Remove tourniquet and apply local anesthetic (Ela-Max, Emla, lidocaine, etc.).
- Place moisture-proof barrier under the arm to prevent blood contamination of the bed linens during procedure.
- Cleanse the potential insertion site according to institution policy. Using a circular motion and friction, clean an area of 3 to 4 inches in diameter. Allow prepping solution to dry completely to maximize bacteriocidal action. Bacteriocidal action occurs only while solution is wet.
- Apply a tourniquet about 4 inches above the selected venipuncture site.
- Stabilize the vein by placing thumb on the vein below the insertion site and pulling the skin down away from the insertion site. The vein will flatten some but remain engorged below the skin. If the vein is not properly stabilized, insertion will be difficult. The thumb should be out of the insertion path. If you have to insert the cannula over the thumb, the angle of penetration will be too steep and there is a strong possibility that the catheter will go through the back wall of the vein.
- Holding the flashback chamber (not the hub) with the needle bevel up and the catheter pointing in the direction of blood flow, pierce the skin on top of the vein at an angle only high enough to enter the vein (15 to 20 degrees), depending on how superficial the vein is (lower for superficial and higher for deeper), and enter the vein in one motion (at least one fourth of catheter length to ensure both stylet and catheter enter vein).

- When blood is visible in the flashback chamber, lower the catheter almost level to the skin, and pull back slightly on the flashback chamber. This pulls the sharp tip back into the catheter (hooding) preventing vein damage. Then slide the catheter and stylet into the vein until the hub is at the insertion site.
- Release the tourniquet.
- While holding the IV catheter with the thumb and index finger of your nondominant hand, place light pressure with the remaining fingers to the vein above the catheter tip. This compression will minimize blood flowing from the catheter when the stylet is removed.
- Remove the stylet with your dominant hand and attach either the cap or primed administration set to the catheter. Discard the stylet in an approved sharps container.
- Check for patency by either flushing the catheter, if not connected to a fluid container, or lowering the fluid container to visualize blood flow back into the tubing. Raise container and attach to IV stand.
- Secure the catheter with tape to minimize movement. Apply dressing over insertion site and catheter but not the hub-administration set connection. Apply additional tape to secure tubing.
- Write the date, time of insertion, length of catheter, and your initials on the dressing.
- Regulate the IV flow to correct the drip rate, or set the electronic monitoring device appropriately.

TAKE HOME POINTS

1. Make sure the IV solution is clear and free of particles.
2. Allow skin prep solutions to completely dry before performing veinipuncture.
3. Select an IV catheter appropriate for the patient's vein size and the prescribed flow rate.
4. Select a site that allows for maximum patient mobility.
5. Do not partially withdraw the stylet from the cannula and then reinsert it. This can result in catheter damage.

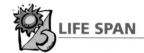

LIFE SPAN

Always use the smallest gauge catheter in the largest vein to minimize vein damage.

Do You UNDERSTAND?

DIRECTIONS: **Select the best answer.**

1. A catheter lock device:
   a. Prohibits patient movement
   b. Is used intermittently
   c. Administers IV fluids continuously
   d. Attaches to a solution container

2. Fluid replacement is necessary:
   a. When the patient is vomiting
   b. When the patient is immobile
   c. When the patient is cold to the touch
   d. When the patient is hypertensive
3. A long-term catheter is:
   a. PICC
   b. Implanted port
   c. Hohn
   d. Pulmonary artery

What IS an Intravenous Gravity Flow Rate?

Total infusion times for large volume solutions are prescribed by the physician or advanced practice nurse and monitored by the health care provider. When an IV infuses by gravity, the *IV flow rate* is determined by counting the number of drops per minute that fall from the drip chamber of the administration set. Drops may be observed and counted by the health care provider as they fall into the drip chamber, or they may be automatically counted by an electronic monitoring device. The number of drops contained in 1 mL of IV fluid are determined by the size of the opening in the drip chamber. Although the size opening varies with the administration set, it is always specified in drops (gtt) per milliliter (mL) on the administration package. Macro (large drop) sets provide either 10 gtt/mL, 15 gtt/mL, or 20 gtt/mL, and the micro (small drop) set provides 60 gtt/mL. The number of drops per milliliter is commonly referred to as the *drop factor.*

An infusion rate that is too fast can result in circulatory overload. This may be life threatening to patients with cardiovascular disease and other disorders.

What You NEED TO KNOW

Three basic factors should be considered when calculating the infusion rate: (1) the total number of hours the IV is to infuse, (2) the drop factor of the administration set, and (3) the total volume of solution to be infused.

To determine how many drops per minute need to be counted, you must know how many milliliters per minute you must infuse. With large-volume infusions, you must first identify the milliliters per hour (total volume ÷ total time). Then you can calculate the milliliters per minute by dividing the hourly milliliter volume by 60 minutes. Using the ratio-proportion method, the left ratio is the drop factor on the administration set package. The right ratio has x (the unknown drop rate) in the numerator and the volume (mL per minute) in the denominator. Calculations are rounded to the nearest milliliter because parts of a drop cannot be counted.

Example: **Dr. Jones has prescribed 1000 mL of D₅W to infuse over 8 hours. The drop factor on administration set is 15 gtt/mL.**

Total volume	Total time	Hourly volume
1000 mL	÷ 8 hr	= 125 mL/hr

Hourly rate		Minute volume
125 mL	÷ 60 min	= 2 mL/min

Drop factor

$$\frac{15 \text{ gtt}}{1 \text{ mL}} = \frac{x \text{ gtt (unkown gtt)}}{2 \text{ mL (minute volume)}} \qquad x = 15 \times 2$$

x = 30 gtt/min

What You DO

To Set the Infusion Rate

- Using the roller clamp, increase or decrease the flow rate to approximate the desired rate.
- Choose a short time interval, such as 15 seconds, and regulate the rate within that time frame. For example, to set the rate at 30 gtt/min, hold a watch with a second hand close to the drip chamber and regulate to 15 drops per 30 seconds. Once you have obtained the desired range, count the drops for 1 minute to ensure accuracy. When using an

electronic monitoring device, follow the manufacturer's instructions to set the desired rate.

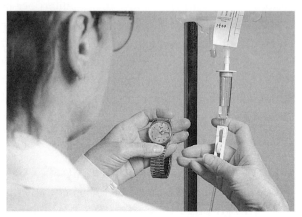

Nurse counting drops. *(From Potter PA, Perry AG: Fundamentals of nursing, ed 6, St Louis, 2005, Mosby.)*

Do You UNDERSTAND?

DIRECTIONS: Fill in the blanks.

1. From time to time you should manually count the drops falling into the drip chamber to _____ _____ of the infusion rate.

2. Count drops for_____ _____ to ensure the correct infusion rate.

DIRECTIONS: Calculate the drops per minute (dpm).

3. You are to administer 500 mL normal saline over 6 hours, and your drop factor is 20 gtt/min. How many gtt/min should the patient receive? _____

Answers: 1. **double check the accuracy; 2. 1 minute; 3. 28 gtt/min (rounded to nearest whole number 27.7 dpm).**

What is Flow Regulation?

Flow regulation is required to allow the health care practitioner the ability to control the flow of fluid from the container to the patient.

What You NEED TO KNOW

Flow Rate Regulation Devices

For fluid to flow a pressure gradient must be present between the fluid container and the patient's IV insertion site. There are three systems available that enable the regulation of fluid flow at different levels of accuracy: gravity, mechanical, and electronic.

Gravity is the simplest. With this system the height of the fluid container above the level of the patient's heart provides the necessary pressure for fluid flow. The atmospheric pressure (PSI) exerted on the fluid container is greater than that of the patient's peripheral veins and central veins and therefore permits flow to occur. For the optimum pressure gradient, the fluid container should be 36 inches above the level of the patient's heart. The lower the bag in relation to the level of the patient's heart, the lower the pressure exerted on the bag and the slower the flow rate. In order to set a flow rate with different container heights, the roller clamp will be more opened or closed. But if the height of the container changes, such as when the bed is raised, the flow rate will slow. Gravity is safe but does not provide consistent accuracy. With manual flow regulators, such as Dial-A-Flow and Control-A-Flow, the flow rate is adjusted by turning a dial to the prescribed flow rate. Accuracy with these systems varies widely and can be impacted by patient activity (the height between the fluid container and the patient varies), vein location, and head height of the solution. In conditions such as fluid overload, right-side heart failure, and pulmonary hypertension, the use of gravity flow as a regulatory system is not recommended.

Mechanical systems, such as elastomeric pumps and the spring-loaded syringe pump, require no electricity. They use a combination of atmospheric pressure and the addition of a resister (adds resistance) to the distal tip of the tubing to deliver a specific flow rate. With these systems, you do not manually set the flow rate. It is determined by the tubing. These pumps are used in home care settings with the ambulatory patient.

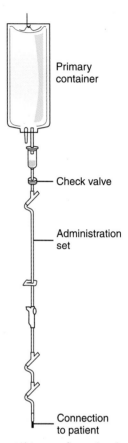

Primary tubing configured to be used with piggybacks. *(Provided by Professional Learning Systems, Inc. Atlanta, GA.)*

Rate accuracy can be altered when there are changes to ambient temperature or pressure, such as infusing the solution cold instead of at room temperature.

Electronic systems require electricity, battery packs, or both, and are accurate, have free-flow prevention systems, and initiate an alarm to sound when problems with the infusion occur. There are two types of electronic systems: nonvolumetric and volumetric. Nonvolumetric devices called *controllers* count drops while using gravity as the pressure source. Volumetric pumps deliver a preset fluid rate over a specific time period using constant force to generate the presssure gradient. The force exerted by the pump is relaed to the resistance generated by the contact of the fluid on the tubing as the fluid moves through the tubing. Pumps are very accurate and are preferred for infusions that require a high level of accuracy, such as with infants, children, and solutions infused through central lines.

Time Tapes

A *time tape* is a strip of tape or a commercially prepared paper strip that is used to monitor an IV container infusing by gravity. Time tapes help you to monitor the infusion over time. At a glance, you can see if the IV is infusing slower or faster than prescribed. For example, a 1000 mL of IV solution that has been prescribed to run over 8 hours should have one half of the total amount (i.e., 500 mL) infused after 4 hours. Using a time tape, the health care provider is able to tell at a glance whether the fluid is on time (time strip line is at the 500 mL mark on the solution bag).

Age-Specific Considerations

There are considerations when administering IV medications to certain age groups.

Infants and children. Because of the danger of accidental overhydration, you must take extreme care when administering IVs to infants and small children. Today, electronic volumetric pumps are required in the pediatric population. You must still monitor the infusion and the insertion site carefully.

Older adults. Remember that your older patients may have decreased renal function. When administering IV fluids and medications, you must be careful not to put the patient at risk of fluid overload. The prolonged clearance of drugs from the body will incease the risk of toxicity. Administration times may need to be adjusted.

TAKE HOME POINTS

- Proper regulation of IV flow is critical to a patient's well-being.
- Flow rates may be regulated manually or by electronic monitoring devices.
  - Do not attempt to "catch up" an IV that is behind schedule.

LIFE SPAN

All pediatric IV solutions and mediations should be delivered by an electronic pump with free flow protection to prevent fluid overload or speed shock. Fluid overload is especially serious in the infant and small child.

An infusion rate that is too slow will have a decreased systemic effect, and it may cause circulatory collapse in individuals who are dehydrated or in shock. Nevertheless, never increase the flow rate to allow an IV to "catch up" without a physician's order.

What You DO

An electronic pump automatically infuses a programmed flow rate. Flow rates are preset by the health care provider. The electronic monitoring device has alarms to alert the health care provider that the pump is not programmed correctly, or that there is a system problem. Common alarms are *occlusion* (identifies that the preset resistance limit has been surpassed), *air in line* (air bubbles pass through the pumping action), and *upstream alarm* (pump is unable to meet the stroke volume requirement). Some additional pump alarms include "infusion complete," "low battery" or "low power," "not infusing," "nonfunctional," and "door open." Because the pump does not detect infiltration or a disconnection when the fluid continues to flow, you must check your patient's IV sites and connections on a regular basis.

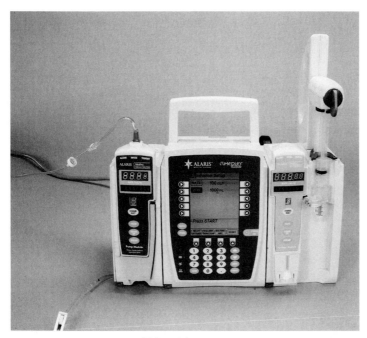

Volumetric pump.

Do You UNDERSTAND?

DIRECTIONS: **Match the terms in Column A with the corresponding descriptions in Column B.**

Column A

1. _____ Required in the pediatiric patient.

2. _____ Nonelectronic monitoring

3. _____ Check drops/gtt

4. _____ IV infusion behind schedule

Column B

a. To confirm prescribed infusion rate and children and disconnections

b. electronic pump

c. Never "catch up" infusion

d. Time tapes

What IS Titration?

Titration is the term used when IV fluids are regulated to provide a specific amount of drug within a given time period based on prescribed parameters. Titration is used in critical-care situations and in specialty areas, such as obstetrics and pediatrics.

What You NEED TO KNOW

Titrating a medication is giving more or less of a medication based on assessment parameters. Each medication has drug-specific information that you need to know, including the onset of the medication, peak effect, medication antagonist, time frame for reassessment, and consequences of sudden medication withdrawal. Titration prescriptions should include the purpose for titrating (i.e., chest pain) and a maximum dose. From this information, a titration table that includes increments of both

Answers: 1. b; 2. d; 3. a; 4. c.

intravenous infusion rate and drug dosage is calculated and kept on the intravenous pump for easy access. Increments are determined by the relationship of dose to patient response. Usually, if the dose range is small, increments are small. If the dose range is wider, then the increments are larger. Most titration prescriptions also include parameters (i.e., blood pressure, respiratory rate, pulse rate, temperature, or level of consciousness), or parameters are found in specific facility protocols. Typically the administration consists of a dose per unit of time—either in mcg/min, mg/min, mg/hr, Units/hr, mg/kg/hr, or mcg/kg/minute. However, electronic pumps require milliliters per hour for programming. Titration calculations often need conversions for both time and units of measure.

What You DO

Titration calculations may be performed using ratio-proportion.

Example: **Start nitroglycerin IV (NTG) at 20 micrograms/minute (mcg/min) for chest pain for acute myocardial infarction (AMI) and titrate for chest pain to maximum 90 mcg/min and also keep systolic blood pressure >100 mm Hg. You have 250 mL NS with 50 mg of nitroglycerin.**

Step 1: Convert mcg to mg.
  20 mcg = 0.02 mg (remember that you drop zeros to the right of the last digit to right of decimal point).

Step 2: Convert milligrams per minute to milligrams per hour by multiplying by 60.

$$0.02 \text{ mg} \times 60 \text{ min} = 1.2 \text{ mg/hr}$$

Step 3: Set up ratio-proportion to identify mL/hr.

$$\frac{50 \text{ mg}}{250 \text{ mL}} = \frac{1.2 \text{ mg}}{x \text{ mL}}$$

$$50 \times x = 1.2 \times 250$$

$$50x = 300 \qquad x = 300 \div 50$$

$$x = 6 \text{ mL/hr}$$

Develop a titration chart using 10-mcg increments.

$$\frac{20 \text{ mcg}}{6 \text{ mL}} = \frac{30 \text{ mcg}}{x \text{ mL}} \text{ (10-mcg increase) } 20 \text{ x} = 180 \quad \text{x} = 180 \div 20$$
$$\text{x} = 9 \text{ mL/hr}$$

$$\frac{20 \text{ mcg}}{6 \text{ mL}} = \frac{40 \text{ mcg}}{x \text{ mL}} \text{ (10-mcg increase) } 20 \text{ x} = 240 \quad \text{x} = 240 \div 20$$
$$\text{x} = 12 \text{ mL/hr}$$

$$\frac{20 \text{ mcg}}{6 \text{ mL}} = \frac{50 \text{ mcg}}{x \text{ mL}} \text{ (10-mcg increase) } 20 \text{ x} = 300 \quad \text{x} = 300 \div 20$$
$$\text{x} = 15 \text{ mL/hr}$$

$$\frac{20 \text{ mcg}}{6 \text{ mL}} = \frac{60 \text{ mcg}}{x \text{ mL}} \text{ (10-mcg increase) } 20 \text{ x} = 360 \quad \text{x} = 360 \div 20$$
$$\text{x} = 18 \text{ mL/hr}$$

$$\frac{20 \text{ mcg}}{6 \text{ mL}} = \frac{70 \text{ mcg}}{x \text{ mL}} \text{ (10-mcg increase) } 20 \text{ x} = 420 \quad \text{x} = 420 \div 20$$
$$\text{x} = 21 \text{ mL/hr}$$

$$\frac{20 \text{ mcg}}{6 \text{ mL}} = \frac{80 \text{ mcg}}{x \text{ mL}} \text{ (10-mcg increase) } 20 \text{ x} = 480 \quad \text{x} = 480 \div 20$$
$$\text{x} = 24 \text{ mL/hr}$$

$$\frac{20 \text{ mcg}}{6 \text{ mL}} = \frac{90 \text{ mcg}}{x \text{ mL}} \text{ (10-mcg increase) } 20 \text{ x} = 540 \quad \text{x} = 540 \div 20$$
$$\text{x} = 27 \text{ mL/hr}$$

When the drop factor is 60 gtt/mL, the milliliters per hour is the same as the drops per minute.

TAKE HOME POINTS

The health care provider is responsible for knowing whether a titrated drug is in a safe dose range for a particular patient. If in doubt, consult the *Physician's Desk Reference, Mosby's Gen Rx,* or the prescribing professional.

Do You UNDERSTAND?

DIRECTIONS: **Calculate the milligrams per hour.**

1. The prescription is to give 1 g aminophylline in 500 mL D_5W over 10 hours. How many milligrams per hour will the patient receive?_____

DIRECTIONS: **Fill in the blanks.**

2. To titrate up, you _____ the drug rate.

3. Titration dose is based on the _____ _____ of the patient's body weight.

What IS an Intravenous Piggyback?

An *IV piggyback* (IVPB) is a small volume bag that holds 50 to 250 mL of solution. Small volume infusions can be administered alone but are commonly added (piggybacked) to a primary solution. Total solution volume and total infusion time are found on the pharmacy label, not the prescription.

What You NEED TO KNOW

The infusion time is commonly written in minutes not hours. Because pump programming requires time in hours, when using a pump, the total number of minutes must be converted to its hour decimal equivalent before the ratio-proportion method can be used to determine the rate. Some equivalents are simple, such as 30 minutes is 0.5 hours. If you do not know what the decimal equivalent is, you can always determine it by using the ratio-proportion method. The left ratio is 60 min/hr and the right ratio is the minute rate (on pharmacy label)/x hr. Then the solution volume can be divided by the hourly decimal equivalent to determine mL/hr. An IVPB is connected to the primary solution administration set by a short secondary administration set. The set is attached to the highest y-site port of a primary set configured with a back-check valve. This valve allows the primary fluid to flow but prevents the secondary fluid from flowing into the primary fluid. Piggyback medications usually come premixed from the pharmacy. (When they are not premixed, you should follow the manufacturer's instructions carefully.) Secondary fluids and medications must be compatible with primary fluids. Some drugs specify that they should be attached to the y-site nearest the insertion site.

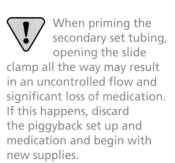

When priming the secondary set tubing, opening the slide clamp all the way may result in an uncontrolled flow and significant loss of medication. If this happens, discard the piggyback set up and medication and begin with new supplies.

Answers: **2. increase; 3. milligrams per kilogram.**

What You DO

- Check the prescription, check for compatibility of medication, and explain the IVPB procedure to the patient and his or her family.
- Calculate mL/hr.
- Gather supplies (medication bag, secondary IV tubing, metal hook, alcohol, "needleless connector").
- Check the IV solution for clarity, and inspect the IV site for signs of inflamation, swelling, or pain. Restart the IV in a new site if any of these are present.
- Spike the IVPB bag and prime tubing. This is accomplished by either opening the slide clamp slightly and filling the tubing (difficult to control) or, after spiking with the slide clamp closed, attach to the appropriate y-site. Lower the IVPB bag and open the slide clamp. Fluid from the primary container will fill the secondary tubing and drip chamber half. Close the clamp, raise the IVBP bag, and attach to the IV pole.
- Attach the metal hook to a different spot on the IV pole and attach the primary solution to the hook. The IVPB will be higher than the primary IV. Open the slide clamp on the IVPB tubing completely. Adjust flow rate using the primary set roller clamp. Note that while the IVBP is infusing no drops are falling in the primary solution drip chamber. Once the IVPB solution is complete, the primary solution will begin to flow again.
- Once the IVPB infusion is complete, readjust the infusion rate to the primary rate. It may be necessary to remove the hook and return the primary solution to the original head height.
- If using an electronic monitoring or pumping device, set it up according to the manufacturer's directions. IVPBs are referred to as secondary on the pump display. Even with a pump, the secondary fluid must be placed higher than the primary fluid.

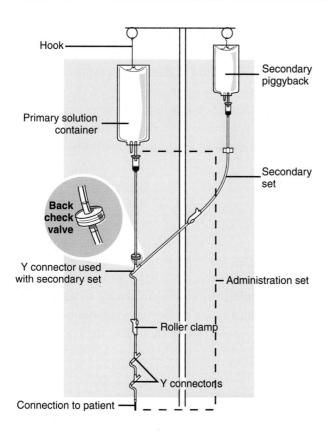

Hook

Primary solution container

Back check valve

Y connector used with secondary set

Roller clamp

Connection to patient

Secondary piggyback

Secondary set

Administration set

Y connectors

TAKE HOME POINTS

- To eliminate air from the administration set tubing, prime the secondary tubing by filling it with primary fluid.
- To allow the IVPB to infuse, always lower the primary container below the secondary bag.
- If not using a pump use the roller clamp on the primary line to regulate the IV flow.

Do You UNDERSTAND?

DIRECTIONS: **Select the correct answer.**

1. Which of the following statements about IVPBs is true?
   a. Both solutions (primary and secondary) in an IVPB system are infused at the same time.
   b. The IVPB must be placed higher than the primary solution in order to flow.
   c. If you don't take the piggyback down when it is empty, air will get into the IV.
   d. Piggybacks make it possible to give IV medications without having to start another IV.

2. IVPB systems:
   a. When one solution is being administered continuously, an additional medication or fluid can be infused without starting a second IV.
   b. Are at high risk of developing air bubbles in the line
   c. Never come premixed from the pharmacy
   d. Only allow solutions mixed with D_5W to be infused

What IS an IV Push?

IV push administration is the most effective method of administration for some drugs but also the most hazardous because a concentrated amount of drug is injected into the circulatory system in a short time. With IV push, administration of high concentrations of medication are pushed by syringe through a capped catheter or the low y-site of a primary administration set.

Advantages	Disadvantages
1. Rapid and usually predictable drug response. 2. Ability to closely monitor patient during drug administration.	1. Adverse effects occur at the same rate as therapeutic effects. 2. Speed shock. 3. Phlebitis.

Incorrect placement of the IV catheter may cause irritation of the lining of the blood vessels, resulting in tissue damage or escape of the medication into the tissue (infiltration).

What You NEED TO KNOW

When administering medications using IV push, the IV catheter must be correctly placed in the vein when the medication is given to prevent vein damage or infiltration. The rate of administration of an IV push is calculated based on the volume of medication that can be given each minute. When a specific rate of administration is not given, the standard rate is 1 mL/min.

Answers: 2, a.

What You DO

IV Push Administration with a Primary Administration Set with a Peripheral Catheter

- Check the prescription for medication order, time, dose, and route.
- Identify the patient.
- Gather supplies (the IV drug, diluted as directed by manufacturer; two 3-mL syringes with saline solution; an alcohol wipe; and a watch with a second hand).
- Explain the procedure to the patient and family members.
- Wash your hands and put on clean gloves.
- Check the site for signs of infection or infiltration. (If a problem is noted, initiate a new site.)
- Swab the y-site closest to the patient with an alcohol wipe.
- Attach syringe containing the saline to the y-site.
- Pinch the IV tubing immediately above the y-site to temporarily stop the flow of IV solution.
- Slowly flush catheter with saline flush while palpating above the catheter tip for signs of cool skin temperature and swelling. If the patient complains of burning stop. Reposition arm and attempt again. If burning persists, the safest intervention is to discontinue the IV and restart in another location.
- Attach the syringe with the medication and administer medication at the prescribed rate. (Use your watch to time the injection rate.)
- Attach the second saline syringe and flush slowly to clear the tubing of any residual medication and move the medication into the main circulation.
- Remove the syringe, release the IV tubing, and allow the IV solution to flow at the prescribed rate.
- Document the administration of the medication.
- Observe the patient for medication effects and for adverse reactions.

IV Push Administration with a Central Venous Catheter

With IV push administration through a central vein, the procedure of saline flush, medication administration, saline flush is the same as with the peripheral catheter. However, with a central venous catheter, improper administration can cause catheter damage. First it is important to open the clamp on the extension prior to applying pressure to the syringe plunger. Commonly the saline flush before and after medication administration uses a 10 mL volume. The greatest danger can occur with the application of too much force on the plunger of the syringe during the flush or medication injection actions. Because central venous catheters are longer than peripheral catheters, you may feel increased resistance. It is important to not overcome resistance with increased pressure. If resistance is felt, stop and reposition the patient, then have the patient cough and take deep breath. Then try to flush again. The final saline flush is very important. Clearing the catheter of medication prevents the possibility of precipitate formation in the catheter. When disengaging the syringe, you need to know what type of cap is being used (nonpositive pressure versus positive pressure). When positive pressure caps are used, the syringe is disengaged before the clamp is closed. When nonpositive pressure caps are used, pressure is maintained on the syringe plunger, the clamp is closed, and then the syringe is removed.

Do You UNDERSTAND?

DIRECTIONS: **Select the correct answer.**

1. Before administering a IV push medication you check the patient's IV site and notice redness and slight swelling. You should:
   a. Inject a small amount of saline and see if the swelling increases.
   b. Select a new site and insert a new IV line.
   c. Continue to observe the site and obtain an order to give the medication by mouth.
   d. Discontinue the IV and give the medication IM.

DIRECTIONS: **Fill in the blanks.**

2. IV push is the most _____ method of drug administration, but it is also the most _____.
3. Incorrect placement of the catheter may cause irritation of the lining of the blood vessels, resulting in _____ _____.

Answers: 1. b; 2. effective, dangerous; 3. tissue damage.

References

Curren A, Munday L: *Math for meds,* ed 9, San Diego, 2004, WI Publications.

Leahy JM, Kizalay PE: *Foundations of nursing practice: a nursing process approach,* Philadelphia, 1998, WB Saunders.

Macklin D, Chernecky C: *Real world survival guide: IV therapy,* St Louis, 2004, WB Saunders.

Macklin D, Chernecky C, Infortuna H: *Math for clinical practice,* St Louis, 2005, Mosby.

Morris, DG: *Calculate with confidence,* ed 3, St Louis, 2002, Mosby.

Pickar GD: *Dosage calculations,* ed 7, Albany, NY, 2004, Delmar.

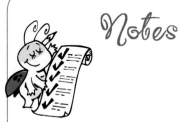

Notes

NCLEX® Review

Circle the correct answer.

1. The major purpose of an IV to keep vein open (KVO) is to:
   1 Provide continuous fluid intake over a long period.
   2 Provide a route for continuous admitnistration of IV medication.
   3 Provide immediate access to the venous system, if necessary.
   4 Ensure adequate hydration in a dehydrated patient.

2. Before inserting an IV device, a tourniquet should be applied:
   1 About 2 inches above the selected site
   2 About 4 inches above the selected site
   3 No more than 1 inch above the selected site
   4 At any point on the extremity, as long as it is above the selected site

3. IV needles should be inserted at an angle of about:
   1 20 degrees
   2 30 degrees
   3 45 degrees
   4 Flush with the skin

4. The IV drip factor is the:
   1 Actual rate at which the IV should flow
   2 Amount per hour that a patient receives
   3 Number of drops per milliliter
   4 Milliliters per minute that a patient receives

5. The reason an IV bolus is the most dangerous route of medication administration is because:
   1 Larger amounts of the drug are given by this route than by any of the other routes.
   2 The drug remains in the body for a longer period.
   3 Results are unpredictable.

4 A concentrated amount of drug is injected into the circulatory system in a short time.

Directions: Calculate drops per minute (gtt/min) and round rates to nearest whole number.

6. Prescription: Infuse D_5W NS at 125 mL/hr (drop factor of tubing 60 gtt/mL).
   mL/min _____ gtt/min _____

7. Prescription: Infuse D_5W 1000 mL at 100 mL/hr (drop factor of tubing 15 gtt/mL).
   mL/min _____ gtt/min _____

8. Prescription: Infuse gentamicin 70 mg every 8 hours. Rate 200 mL/hr (drip factor 60 gtt/mL).
   mL/min _____ gtt/min _____

9. Prescription: Infuse D_5NS 2000 mL intravenous over 20 hr (drop factor 10 gtt/mL).
   mL/min _____ gtt/min _____

10. Prescription: Infuse D_5 ½ NS intravenous at 80 mL/hr (drop factor 20 gtt/mL).
    mL/min _____ gtt/min _____

True or False

11. Electronic pumps alarm to notify you of an infiltration.

12. Patient activity impacts gravity flow rates.

13. Piggyback medications must be attached to primary sets that have a back-check valve.

14. When resistance is felt while flushing a central line, it is appropriate to apply additional pressure with your thumb to administer the IV push medication.

15. Flow rate accuracy can be altered when there are changes to ambient temperature when using a mechanical system.

NCLEX® Review Answers

1. **3** An IV that is intended to keep the vein open is run at a very slow rate, but it provides immediate venous access should it be necessary for emergency drug or fluid administration. It is not intended to deliver continuous fluid intake over a long period or continuous medication. A dehydrated person will need continuous fluids at a much faster rate than the rate necessary to keep the vein open.

2. **2** The appropriate distance to place a tourniquet to obstruct venous flow and distend the vein is 4 to 6 inches. Placing it 2 inches above the selected site is too close to the site to obstruct venous flow and distend the vein adequately. Placing it 1 inch is too close to the site and could hinder the nurse's effort to access the vein. Placing it at any point could result in it being too close and interfering with insertion or being too far away to affect the selected site.

3. **2** A 30-degree angle is the correct angle at which to properly access a vein. A 20-degree angle is insufficient, and a 45-degree angle is too steep and often results in going through the vein.

4. **3** The IV drip factor is the actual size of the opening through which the IV drips. It varies by manufacturer and is always stated on the tubing package. The drip factor is not the rate at which the IV should flow, although it is a factor in calculation of the flow rate. The drip factor is also not the amount per hour that a patient should receive or the number of milliliters per minute that the patient should receive, although the drip factor is part of the calculation to determine how many milliliters are given.

5. **4** The IV bolus is the most dangerous route of medication administration because a concentrated amount of drug is injected into the circulatory system in a short time. The patient may have an exaggerated response that requires emergency attention. *Smaller,* rather than larger, amounts of a drug are usually given IV because the drug gets into the circulatory system immediately (in contrast to drugs given IM or SQ). A drug administered by IV bolus has an immediate effect and is likely to remain in the body for a *shorter* period as compared with a drug administered by other routes. Results from an IV bolus are not always predictable, but the immediate entrance into the circulatory system is the reason it is the most dangerous method.

6.   2.1 mL/min; 125 gtt/min.

7.   1.7 mL/min; 26 gtt/min.

8.   3.3 mL/min; 200 gtt/min.

9.   1.7 mL/min; 17 gtt/min.

10.   1.3 mL/min; 26 gtt/min.

11.   False. Electronic pumps sound an alarm when the preset resistance limit has been surpassed.

12.   True. Patient activity impacts gravity flow rates.

13.   True. Piggyback medications must be attached to primary sets that have a back-check valve so that the piggyback medication cannot flow into the primary fluid.

14.   False. Applying increased resistance can damage the catheter.

15.   True. Mechanical system infusion rates can be altered with changes to ambient temperature or pressure.

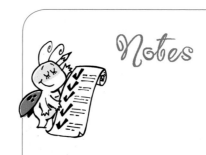

13 Intravenous Additives

What You WILL LEARN

After reading this chapter, you will know how to do the following:

- ✔ List five common intravenous additives.
- ✔ Calculate intravenous rates of intravenous fluids with additives based on clinical patient needs and prescription. List steps required to administer IV additives.

What IS an Intravenous Additive?

Intravenous (IV) additives are medications that are added to an IV solution and administer continuously over a specified period. The medication may be added to the IV solution before administration, or it may be added while the IV is infusing.

What You NEED TO KNOW

Most IV additives are potent medications, so diluting them in large volume IV solution is the safest method of administration. You must always check the compatibility of a medication with the IV solution in which it is to be diluted or with other medications already added to the IV solution.

What You DO

To Administer IV Additives:

- Check the prescription and the medication label.
- Ask the patient about medication allergies and check the chart.
- Examine the medication label and double check that it is intended for IV use.
- Consider the Six Rights of Medication Administration (right medication, right dose, right patient, right time, right route, and right documentation).
- Determine safe dose range for the medication and notify the prescribing professional if the medication is out of dose range for your patient.
- Check the patient's identification band, and explain the procedure to the patient and family members.
- Gather supplies (medication to be added to the IV container; 10 to 20 mL syringe; 19- to 21-gauge, 1½-inch needle; diluent compatible with the medication; IV solution; alcohol wipe; and medication label).
- Prepare the medication according to the manufacturer's instructions.
- Locate the medication injection port on the IV container, and swab it with an alcohol wipe.
- Insert the needle into the center of the medication port and inject the medication.
- Gently agitate the container, and turn it end to end to mix the medication.
- Fill out the medication label, noting the name of the medication, the dose, the date, the time it was added, and your initials.
- Place the label upside down on the IV container.

   If the IV is not infusing or complications (infiltration, phlebitis) are present, restart the IV according to the protocol used by your medical facility. If the IV is infusing properly, check the IV site, tubing connections, and rate of flow before administering additives. You must also remember to check the IV solution for compatibility of medication additive and solution before administration.

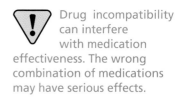

Drug incompatibility can interfere with medication effectiveness. The wrong combination of medications may have serious effects.

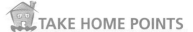

TAKE HOME POINTS

- Check for compatibility of drug additives and the IV solution (and any medications already in the IV solution) before administering an IV additive.
- Consider any age-related concerns before administering an IV additive.

Age-Specific Considerations

There are also certain considerations when administering IV additives to certain age groups:

Infants and children. To prevent overhydrating an infant or child, always administer large volumes of fluid using an electronic pump. Before adding medications or supplements of any kind to a younger patient's IV, always calculate the safe dose range based on the child's weight. Be sure to notify the prescribing professional if the dose is out of range.

Pregnant women. If the patient is pregnant, consult a pharmacology reference for administration guidelines before injecting IV additives. Failing to do so could harm the fetus.

Older adults. When administering IV additives to older adults, consult a pharmacology reference to check the safety of the medication in patients that may have decreased liver and kidney function. If necessary, notify the prescribing professional before administering the medication.

Specific Additives

A few additives are administered on a regular basis. These include multi-vitamin preparations, potassium chloride, magnesium sulfate, sodium bicarbonate, and insulin.

Do You UNDERSTAND?

DIRECTIONS: **You are likely to encounter the words in the puzzle in your work. Circle as many as you can. The words run left to right, right to left, up, down, or diagonally. The words are listed under the puzzle.**

A	R	R	H	Y	T	H	M	I	A	X	G	Z	Y	R	C
Z	D	E	L	B	I	T	A	P	M	O	C	R	F	B	I
S	O	D	I	U	M	F	W	X	Y	Z	T	S	A	L	T
T	S	X	I	Z	Y	Q	P	C	N	I	Z	Q	X	M	Y
W	E	Z	X	T	Y	V	Z	H	O	S	P	I	T	A	L
X	C	A	R	D	I	A	C	L	P	Q	Z	X	N	G	O
E	T	U	L	O	S	V	S	O	K	X	Z	E	F	N	C
M	E	D	I	C	I	N	E	R	D	Q	E	P	Z	E	O
U	X	A	Q	A	P	Q	Z	I	F	D	X	T	E	S	T
I	Z	N	X	N	F	D	X	D	L	Q	A	Z	J	I	X
S	Q	G	Z	N	R	I	Y	E	C	A	L	C	I	U	M
S	P	E	Q	U	F	U	Z	Q	X	P	L	A	W	M	U
A	Z	R	G	L	Q	L	V	X	Y	W	E	R	F	Q	R
T	W	Q	Z	A	B	F	K	E	T	A	R	B	X	A	E
O	Y	I	N	S	U	L	I	N	Y	X	G	O	Q	Z	S
P	I	G	G	Y	B	A	C	K	Z	Q	Y	N	P	F	G

additive   dose   piggyback
allergy   drug   potassium
arrhythmia   fluid   rate
calcium   gram   salt
cannula   hospital   serum
carbon   insulin   sodium
cardiac   IV   solute
chloride   magnesium   test
compatible   medicine   tocolytic
danger   needle   zinc

Multivitamins are incompatible with the following medications:
- Penicillin-G
- Erythromycin
- Tetracycline
- Lincomycin
- Kanamycin
- Streptomycin
- Doxycycline

What IS a Multivitamin Preparation?

A multivitamin preparation is used to prevent and treat vitamin deficiency in patients who cannot ingest food or fluids by mouth or who are receiving their primary nourishment intravenously. Vitamins for IV use are packaged under trade names such as Berocca Parenteral, MVC 93, and MVI Pediatric. Multivitamin products for IV administration are compatible with the most IV solutions (e.g., NS, D_5W, D_5/NS, LR, D_5LR) and are prepared to be administered in 500 mL to 1000 mL of IV solution.

What You NEED TO KNOW

When adding a multivitamin preparation to an IV solution containing other medications, you should check compatibility with the hospital formulary or pharmacy before administering. If the patient is receiving incompatible medications by IV piggyback (IVPB), the medications will have to be administed intermittently instead of piggy back. This way the catheter can be flushed before and after the medication is given and then the continuous infusion can be reattached and begun again.

What You DO

To Administer a Multivitamin Preparation

- Follow the steps for administering IV additives described earlier in this chapter.
- Be sure to note any age-related concerns before administering the medication.
- Always check for compatibility of the IV solution and medication additives.

Do You UNDERSTAND?

DIRECTIONS: **Fill in the blanks.**

1. Patients who cannot take food or fluids _____,
   or are receiving their primary nourishment by IV, need
   supplementary vitamins.
2. Multivitamins are _____
   with the following medications: penicillin-G, erythromycin,
   tetracycline, lincomycin, kanamycin, _____,
   and doxycycline.

What IS Potassium Chloride?

Potassium chloride (KCL) is responsible for the regulation of cellular water balance, electrical conduction in muscle cells, and acid-base balance. In healthy individuals, KCL is supplied by food intake, and regulated by the kidneys. However, some people need to receive KCL supplements. These supplements are commercially prepared as IV additives (e.g., acetate, chloride, and potassium salts) and are used to correct hypokalemia (i.e., low blood potassium levels).

The most common cause of hypokalemia is treatment with thiazide or loop diuretics. However, low levels of potassium may also occur as the result of diarrhea, vomiting, excessive sweating, and strenuous dieting.

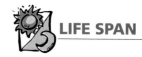 **LIFE SPAN**

Adults should not receive more than 150 mEq/day of KCL. The dose of KCL a child receives is based on the child's body weight in kilograms. The recommended dose of KCL is 20 mEq/hr for adults and 3 mEq/kg/day for children when diluted in a 1000 mL IV solution.

Because patients with hypokalemia also experience reduced levels of chloride, KCL supplements are preferred over potassium supplements. KCL is administered to maintain a blood potassium level between 3 and 5 mEq/L.

What You NEED TO KNOW

Intravenous potassium can be fatal if given inappropriately. Potassium is never given IV push but is always diluted in IV solution. Because of fatal accidents, it is recommended that commercially prepared solutions with potassium already added be used whenever possible. Adding potassium to fluids used to be more common than today. Most often potassium will be admixed in the pharmacy. In rare instances in critical care or emergency areas, potassium may still be admixed. Extreme caution should be used if this arises.

What You DO

To Administer KCL:

- Assess the patient's renal function prior to administration
- Infusion guidelines: 5 to 10 mEq/hr diluted in continuous IV solution 10 mEq to 20 mEq/hr in extreme hypokalemia. Patient must be monitored by ECG.
- Potassium infusions commonly cause pain along the vein. Slowing the infusion (if possible) and applying heat over the vein may lessen the pain.
- Potassium infiltrations can cause tissue sloughing (extravasation) especially with higher concentrations.

Do You UNDERSTAND?

DIRECTIONS: **Label the following statements *True* or *False*.**
1. _____ Potassium chloride must always be diluted prior to intravenous administration.
2. _____ Using commercially available solutions with the potassium already added is preferable to admixing.
3. _____ Potassium infusions can cause pain over the vein.
4. _____ Never give undiluted potassium chloride IV push.

What IS Magnesium Sulfate?

Magnesium sulfate is an anticonvulsant. It is given IV for three reasons:
1. To control seizures in pregnancy-induced hypertension
2. To stop preterm labor as a tocolytic medication
3. To treat and prevent hypomagnesemic states

What You NEED TO KNOW

To use magnesium sulfate to prevent or control seizures in pregnancy-induced hypertension, the patient should receive 4 g to 6 g IV 250 mL D_5W. Keep in mind that IV infusion should not exceed 3 mL of magnesium sulfate per minute; the initial dose may be followed by an infusion of 1 g to 4 g per hour. Although the prescribed dose will vary based on the condition of the patient, the daily dose should not exceed 30 g to 40 g. Patients being treated for hypomagnesemia should receive 5 g of magnesium sulfate IV, diluted. The solution should be infused slowly over 3 hours.

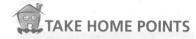

TAKE HOME POINTS

Magnesium sulfate is a potentially dangerous medication.
   Emergency medications and equipment should be available when administering magnesium sulfate.
   It is necessary to check your patient regularly for deep-tendon reflexes (DTRs), which may indicate toxicity before it is apparent in the serum.
   Magnesium sulfate is prepared in grams (g) not grains (gr).

Magnesium sulfate should not be administered unless calcium gluconate is readily available. Calcium gluconate and calcium gluceptate is the antidote for magnesium sulfate, and it should be kept at the bedside along with resuscitation equipment.

What You DO

To Administer Magnesium Sulfate

- Follow the steps for administering IV additives as described earlier in this chapter.
- Check the prescription and medication label carefully. Magnesium sulfate is sometimes ordered in milliequivalents (mEq), although the medication is packaged in grams. Check with the prescribing professional or pharmacist to clarify any discrepancies.
- The patient's serum magnesium level should be checked to determine whether a therapeutic or a toxic level has been reached. If the patient develops any toxicity symptoms, you should notify the physician immediately.
- Patients should be monitored for deep tendon reflex (DTR). Absent DTR indicates toxicity before it is apparent in the serum.
- Signs of toxicity begin at a serum concentration at or above 5 mEq/L.

Signs of Magnesium Sulfate Toxicity

• Flushing	• Respiratory depression
• Hypotension	• Decreased heart rate
• Sweating	• Cardiac dysrhythmias
• Depressed reflexes	• Central nervous system depression
• Flaccid paralysis	• Circulatory collapse

Do You UNDERSTAND?

1. Susan Smith is 29 weeks pregnant and has been admitted to the obstetrics unit with pregnancy-induced hypertension. To prevent seizures, her physician has ordered magnesium sulfate 4 g IV, 250 mL D$_5$W now, followed by magnesium sulfate 2 g/hr. After 2 hours, her pulse is 56 min, her respirations are 14 min, and her face is flushed. Your best action is to:

   a. Slow the infusion and notify the laboratory to draw a magnesium serum level.

b. Check her DTRs and, if normal, continue the IV at the same rate.
c. Discontinue the IV because she is showing signs of toxicity.
d. Stop the magnesium sulfate, keep veins open (KVO) with D_5W, and notify her physician immediately.

What IS Sodium Bicarbonate?

Sodium bicarbonate is a medication used in the treatment of metabolic acidosis and cardiac arrest. This medication increases plasma bicarbonate, which buffers hydrogen ion concentration and reverses acidosis. In emergency settings, it may be administered as an IV push, then given as an IV additive in D_5W solution.

TAKE HOME POINTS
- Sodium bicarbonate is used to reverse acidosis.
- Blood pH and carbon dioxide levels need to be monitored carefully when the patient is receiving sodium bicarbonate.

What You NEED TO KNOW

The dose of sodium bicarbonate that a patient receives is based on body weight in kilograms. In cardiac arrest, for adults and children, a bolus of 1 mEq/kg is given; then 0.5 mEq/kg may be repeated every 5 minutes. Any additional doses should be based on arterial blood gas results.

In metabolic acidosis, adults and children may be given an IV infusion of 2 to 5 mEq/kg over 4 to 8 hours, depending upon blood pH and carbon dioxide levels. Caution must be exercised to prevent excessive elevation of plasma pH because rapid conversion from acidosis to alkalosis can be hazardous to the patient. Because of the high sodium content of sodium bicarbonate, care must also be taken to prevent hypernatremia (i.e., excessive sodium in the blood).

Age-Specific Considerations

There are certain things to consider when using sodium bicarbonate to treat certain age groups:

Infants and children. You should verify the safety of sodium bicarbonate administered to your younger patients based on their body weight. IV infusions to infants should not exceed 8 mEq/day, based on arterial blood gases.

Answers: 1. d.

Pregnant women. If the patient is pregnant, you should consult a pharmacology reference for administration guidelines before injecting sodium bicarbonate.

Older adults. If an older patient is to receive sodium bicarbonate, you should monitor his or her blood levels closely (because of decreased kidney function).

⚠️ Infiltration may cause chemical cellulitis, necrosis, ulceration, or sloughing. Confirm vein patency before administration.

What You DO

To Administer Sodium Bicarbonate

- Follow the steps for administering IV additives as described earlier in this chapter.
- Be sure to note any age-related concerns before administering the medication.

⚠️ Flush IV thoroughly after administration. Sodium bicarbonate is incompatible with many drugs.

Do You UNDERSTAND?

DIRECTIONS: **Fill in the blanks.**

1. Sodium bicarbonate increases _____
_____, which buffers hydrogen ion concentration and reverses acidosis.

2. In metabolic acidosis, care must also be taken to prevent _____
_____
because of the high sodium content of sodium bicarbonate.

What IS Insulin?

Insulin is a substance that lowers blood glucose by increasing transport into the cells and promoting the conversion of glucose to glycogen. Its primary use is to control the blood sugar level in diabetic patients. Although most insulin used to treat diabetes is extracted from beef or pork pancreas, there are also semisynthetic insulins available. Few differences exist among these synthetic insulins and purified pork insulin.

Answers: **1. plasma bicarbonate; 2. hypernatremia.**

However, allergic reactions occur in some patients. Only regular insulin (e.g., Iletin, Humulin) may be given IV. Regular insulin is short acting and provides an immediate, although short-term, effect. Other types of insulin (e.g., Lente, neutral protamine hagedorn [NPH]) are prepared as suspensions that create a longer-lasting effect, but they cannot be given IV. Often a combination of these two types of insulin (e.g., 70/30 insulin) is given to provide both immediate and long-range effects.

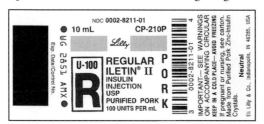

Regular Iletin II label. *Copyright Eli Lilly and Co. All rights reserved.*

> Regular insulin is the only insulin that is suitable for IV use. All other insulins consist of particles in suspension, and these products cannot be given IV. In ketoacidosis, regular insulin may be given IV, 5 to 10 Units initially, then 5 Units/hr until the desired blood glucose level is reached. The method of administration should then be switched to subcutaneous injection. As an IV additive, 50 Units of insulin may be added to 500 mL NS. The dose range for adults is 0.1 Units/kg of body weight/hr as a continuous infusion.

What You NEED TO KNOW

Patients receiving IV insulin must have their blood glucose levels monitored at hourly intervals because insulin reactions can cause life-threatening hypoglycemia. Hypoglycemia can be treated with an IV bolus of glucose or with the oral ingestion of sweet fluids, such as cola or orange juice or both.

Patients receiving IV insulin need to have their serum potassium levels monitored because insulin lowers serum potassium levels by promoting potassium uptake into cells. Monitoring serum potassium levels is critical in patients receiving digoxin because insulin can increase the risk of digoxin-induced dysrhythmia.

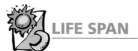

LIFE SPAN

When administering insulin to older adults, consider other medications that may interact, prolong, or shorten the effect of the insulin. Monitor potassium levels carefully if your patient is taking digoxin. Monitor serum levels closely because of decreased kidney function.

What You DO

To Administer IV Insulin

- Check the label carefully to make sure the insulin may be given IV.
- Follow the steps for administering IV additives as described earlier in this chapter.
- Be sure to note any age-related concerns before administering the medication.

TAKE HOME POINTS

- Only regular insulin may be given IV.
- Monitor potassium levels of patients receiving IV insulin.
- Purified pork insulin is almost indistinguishable from human insulin.
- Hourly blood glucose checks are necessary to monitor insulin levels.

Do You UNDERSTAND?

DIRECTIONS: **Match the terms in Column A with the appropriate terms in Column B.**

Column A		Column B
1. _____ Counteract with orange juice		a. Regular insulin
2. _____ Lente		b. Short-acting
3. _____ Only insulin appropriate for IV use		c. NPH insulin
4. _____ Consists of particles in suspension		d. Hypoglycemia
5. _____ Humulin		e. Longer-acting

References

Betz ML, Traw B, Bostrom J: The cost-effectiveness of two intravenous additive systems, *Appl Nurs Res* 7(2):59, 1994.

Curren A, Munday L: *Math for meds,* ed 9, San Diego, 2004, WI Publications.

Gahart BL, Nazareno AR: *2005 intravenous medications. A handbook for nurses and allied health professionals,* ed 21, St Louis, 2002, Mosby.

Gutierrez K: *Pharmacotherapeutics: clinical decision-making in nursing,* Philadelphia, 2000, WB Saunders.

Lilly LA: Magnesium sulfate: is that the right dose? *Am J Nurs* 97(8):12, 1997.

Pickar GD: *Dosage calculations,* ed 7, Albany, NY, 2004, Delmar.

Skidmore RL: *Mosby's drug guide for nurses,* ed 6, St Louis, 2005, Mosby.

Answers: 1. d; 2. e; 3. a; 4. c; 5. b.

NCLEX® Review

Circle the correct answer.

1. The primary reason that many IV additives are given in large amounts of solution is because:
   1 The drugs dissolve better in large amounts of fluid.
   2 The drugs are very potent and are safer when diluted.
   3 The patient is often dehydrated and needs the additional fluid.
   4 Additives in solution are more convenient for the heath care provider.

2. The only type of insulin that may be given IV is:
   1 Long acting
   2 NPH
   3 Regular
   4 Zinc suspension

3. The reason serum potassium must be monitored when a patient is receiving IV potassium is because:
   1 Hyperkalemia is untreatable.
   2 There is a fine line between too little potassium and too much potassium.
   3 Excess potassium can cause life-threatening dysrhythmia.
   4 If hypokalemic, the patient must be treated with insulin.

4. The antidote for magnesium sulfate is:
   1 Calcium gluconate
   2 Calcium carbonate
   3 Calcium citrate
   4 Sodium bicarbonate

5. The physician has prescribed a continuous infusion of sodium bicarbonate in lactated Ringer's solution. You know that this solution is incompatible with sodium bicarbonate. Your best action is to:
   1 Call the pharmacy and ask for a recommendation of a substitute solution.

2 Start the drug in 5% dextrose solution and inform the physician when making rounds.
   3 Start the drug in normal saline and allow it to drip slowly while you try to reach the physician.
   4 Notify the physician.

Fill in the Blanks

6. Multivitamin preparation is used to prevent and treat _____.

7. The most common cause of hypokalemia is treatment with _____.

8. Magnesium sulfate is administered to control _____ _____ in pregnancy-induced hypertension.

9. Patients receiving IV insulin need to have their serum _____ levels monitored.

10. Sodium bicarbonate is used to treat _____ _____.

NCLEX® Review Answers

1. **2** These drugs are potent and will be safer when dissolved in a large amount of solution. Drugs do not necessarily dissolve better in larger amounts of fluid. The primary reason for diluting the drug is not usually the current hydration state of the patient, and the convenience of the health care provider is not a primary factor in this situation.

2. **3** Only regular insulin may be given IV.

3. **3** For this reason, the patient must be closely monitored, and emergency drugs must be kept on hand, because excess potassium can cause life-threatening dysrhythmia. Hyperkalemia is treatable with emergency drugs. A fine line is not

213

what causes concern; rather the seriousness of the effects is the concern. Patients are treated with insulin when they are hyperkalemic.

4. **1** The antidote for magnesium sulfate is calcium gluconate; it should be kept at the bedside when a patient is receiving magnesium sulfate.

5. **4** The physician should be contacted immediately. The pharmacy does not have the right to make this decision; the patient's physician must make the decision. You do not have the order to change the solution and must contact the physician.

6. Multivitamin preparation is used to prevent and treat vitamin deficiency in patients who cannot ingest food or fluids by mouth or are receiving their primary nourishment by IV.

7. The most common cause of hypokalemia is treatment with thiazides or loop diuretics.

8. Magnesium sulfate is administered to control seizures in pregnancy-induced hypertension.

9. Patients receiving IV insulin need to have their serum potassium levels monitored.

10. Sodium bicarbonate is used to treat metabolic acidosis.

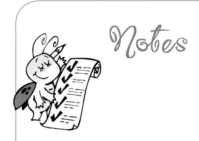

Notes

Special
Medications
and Routes

What You WILL LEARN

After reading this chapter, you will know how to do the following:

✔ Recognize the differences associated with administration of specialty medications.

✔ Calculate dosages to be administered based on patient prescription for medications available in vial and ampule forms.

✔ Calculate appropriate dosages and methods of administration for medications available in patch, inhaler, sublingual, and enteral forms.

✔ Identify prefilled-syringe medications and calculate appropriate dosages based on clinical prescription.

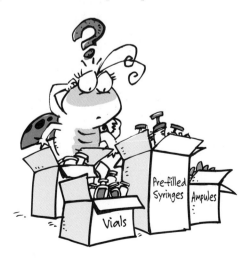

As a health care provider, you will need to be familiar with special medications, such as those packaged in vials, ampules, prefilled syringes, transdermal patches, and inhalers. You will also need to understand that special delivery routes, feeding tubes, and sublingual medications fall into this category.

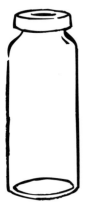

What IS a Vial?

A *vial* is a sealed container of liquid or powdered medication. Vials have rubber stoppers that allow the medication inside to be drawn out (the solute can be withdrawn from the vial through the rubber stopper and mixed with a solvent to create a solution that can be used for a single or multiple dose). Examples of medications supplied in vials are epinephrine, heparin sodium, mannitol, hydroxyzine (Vistaril), phenobarbital sodium, hydrocortisone (Solu-Cortef), gentamicin sulfate (Garamycin), cefazolin sodium (Kefzol), digoxin (Lanoxin), and potassium chloride (KCL).

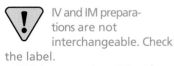
IV and IM preparations are not interchangeable. Check the label.

KCL is never given IV push or bolus. Instead, it should always be added to IV fluid and mixed well. To do this, you must invert the IV bag several times after adding the KCL.

What You Need To KNOW

In most cases a syringe (a 1-cc tuberculin syringe or a 3-cc syringe) is used to extract medication from a vial before it is administered to a patient. When administering medications drawn from a vial for intravenous (IV) or intramuscular (IM) use, keep in mind that many IV or IM doses are one third to one half of the oral dose.

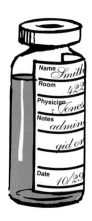

What You DO

- Break up the powder in a vile by gently tapping it against a cushioned surface (you can use your hand, cushioned with a 2 × 4 piece of gauze).
- Remember that with most vials you will need to prepare the correct solute, then add it to the solvent to create the required solution.
- Withdraw the prescribed amount of medication from the vial with a needle and syringe.
- Write the date the vial was opened, the time and date the drug will expire, and your initials on the vial without covering the printed label.
- Write the drug strength on the label (if you mixed a multiple-strength solution).

Age-Specific Considerations

There are also things you should consider when administering certain medications to certain age groups:

Children. The parents of younger patients being treated with corticosteroids (e.g., Solu-Cortef) should be informed that long-term use increases the risk of developing cataracts, osteoporosis, glaucoma, or avascular necrosis of the femur head later in life.

Adults. You should inform your adult patients who receive corticosteroids that these medications can decrease the action of oral contraceptives in women. They also decrease sperm count in men.

Older adults. When working with older patients, keep in mind that the use of corticosteroids increases their risk of hypertension, osteoporosis, and peptic ulcers.

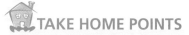

TAKE HOME POINTS

After adding medications to a bag of IV fluid, remember to invert the bag three to four times to distribute the additive evenly.

Reconstitution directions are found on medication labels or package inserts.

For multidose vials, remember to add the same amount of air to the vial as the liquid being taken out. (Doing this will allow you to remove the medication without difficulty.)

Make sure to use the correct diluent or solute (e.g., sterile water, saline, or package-given solute).

Some vials should not be shaken. Shaking decreases the effectiveness of the medication and can cause foaming, which will prevent medication from being drawn out of the vial.

Do You UNDERSTAND?

DIRECTIONS: **Calculate the answers to the following questions.**

1. Jenny is 9 years old and has just arrived in the emergency department with a bee sting. You are asked to immediately give 0.5 mg epinephrine subcutaneously (SC) for anaphylaxis. The epinephrine comes in 30-mg vials at 1 mg/mL. How much epinephrine should you administer? _____

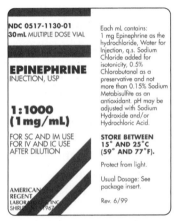

NDC 0517-1130-01
30 mL MULTIPLE DOSE VIAL

Each mL contains:
1 mg Epinephrine as the hydrochloride, Water for Injection, q.s. Sodium Chloride added for isotonicity, 0.5% Chlorobutanol as a preservative and not more than 0.15% Sodium Metabisulfite as an antioxidant. pH may be adjusted with Sodium Hydroxide and/or Hydrochloric Acid.

EPINEPHRINE
INJECTION, USP

**1:1000
(1 mg/mL)**

FOR SC AND IM USE
FOR IV AND IC USE
AFTER DILUTION

**STORE BETWEEN
15° AND 25°C
(59° AND 77°F).**

Protect from light.

Usual Dosage: See package insert.

AMERICAN
REGENT
LABORATORIES INC
SHIRLEY NY 11967

Rev. 6/99

Epinephrine label. *Reproduced with the permission of American Regent Laboratories Inc.*

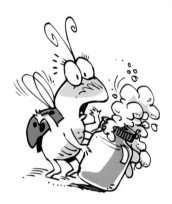

2. Mr. Kwan is 2 days after surgery and has just been diagnosed with a pulmonary embolism. Heparin sodium, 25,000 Units, has been prescribed SC immediately. You have a 10-mL vial of 5000 Units/mL. How much heparin should you give Mr. Kwan? _____

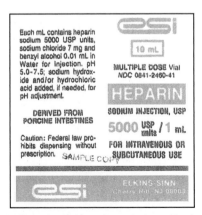

Each mL contains heparin sodium 5000 USP units, sodium chloride 7 mg and benzyl alcohol 0.01 mL in Water for Injection. pH 5.0-7.5; sodium hydroxide and/or hydrochloric acid added, if needed, for pH adjustment.

**DERIVED FROM
PORCINE INTESTINES**

Caution: Federal law prohibits dispensing without prescription. SAMPLE COPY

esi

10 mL

MULTIPLE DOSE Vial
NDC 0641-2460-41

HEPARIN

SODIUM INJECTION, USP

5000 USP units / 1 mL

**FOR INTRAVENOUS OR
SUBCUTANEOUS USE**

esi

ELKINS-SINN
Cherry Hill NJ 08003

Heparin label. *Courtesy Elkins-Sinn Division of America Home Products Corp, Cherry Hill, NJ.*

3. Mrs. Hernendez returns from surgery, and her laboratory electrolyte results state she is low in potassium. The prescription reads, "Give 40 mEq in 500 cc D_5W, over 6 hours." You have a multidose vial of KCL 2 mEq/mL. How much KCL should you draw up into the syringe from the multidose vial? _____

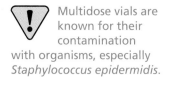

Multidose vials are known for their contamination with organisms, especially *Staphylococcus epidermidis*.

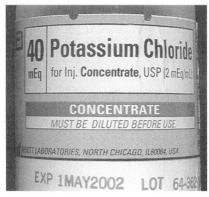

Potassium chloride label. *Reproduced with the permission of Abbott Laboratories.*

4. Debbie is 18 years old and has been brought to the emergency department after a motor vehicle accident (MVA) in which she was thrown through the vehicle's windshield. To reduce her increased intracranial pressure (ICP) and cerebral edema, the physician has prescribed mannitol 2 g/kg. Debbie weighs 68 kg. How many grams will you draw up for infusion? _____

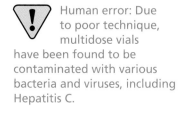

Human error: Due to poor technique, multidose vials have been found to be contaminated with various bacteria and viruses, including Hepatitis C.

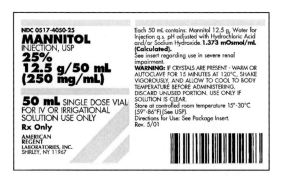

Mannitol label. *Reproduced with the permission of American Regent Laboratories.*

5. Mr. Morgan is going through alcohol withdrawal and is beginning delirium tremens. He is prescribed Vistaril (hydroxyzine) 75 mg IM immediately. You have a 10-ml multidose vial with Vistaril 50 mg/mL. How much Vistaril do you draw up in a syringe? _____

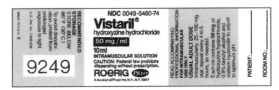

Vistaril label. *Courtesy Pfizer Inc.*

6. James is a 5-year-old child who is often brought to the hospital emergency room with seizures of unknown etiology. He has been prescribed phenobarbital sodium 100 mg. You have a vial of phenobarbital sodium 130 mg/mL in stock. How much phenobarbital do you draw up in a syringe? _____

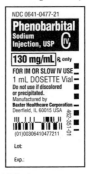

Phenobarbital label. *Courtesy Baxter Healthcare.*

7. Solu-Cortef (hydrocortisone) is prescribed at 100 mg IM now. You have a 4-mL vial of Solu-Cortef 50 mg/mL. How much Solu-Cortef do you draw up into the syringe? _____

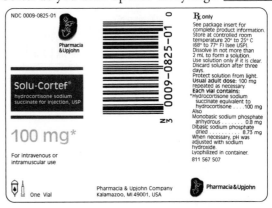

Solu-Cortef label. *Reproduced with the permission of Pharmacia & Upjohn.*

Answers: 5. 1.5 mL; 6. 0.77 or 0.8 mL; 7. 2 mL.

8. Mr. Kronstient has a postoperative infection and is prescribed 60 mg of Garamycin (gentamicin sulfate) to be mixed into a 500-mL bag of D_5W. You have a 20-mL multidose vial with 40 mg/mL. How many milliliters do you draw up into a syringe to mix into the IV bag?_____

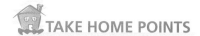

GENTAMICIN SULFATE
Injection, U.S.P.
20 ml Vial
40 mg/ml
For IV use only.

9. Mrs. Soressino has an infection. She has been prescribed Kefzol (cefazolin sodium) 500 mg IV now, and q6h × 7 days. You have a 500-mg vial of Kefzol at 250 mg/mL. How many milliliters do you draw up to mix into Mrs. Soressino's IV bag?_____

CEFAZOLIN SODIUM
Injection, U.S.P.
500 ml Vial
250 mg/ml
For IV use only.

10. Lanoxin (digoxin) 0.025 mg is prescribed. The vial contains 0.25 mg digoxin/mL. How much Lanoxin do you draw up into the syringe?_____

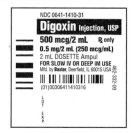

NDC 0641-1410-31
Digoxin Injection, USP
500 mcg/2 mL ℞ only
0.5 mg/2 mL (250 mcg/mL)
2 mL DOSETTE Ampul
FOR SLOW IV OR DEEP IM USE
Mfd. by **Baxter**, Deerfield, IL 60015 USA
462-332-00
(01)00306411410316
L O T
E X P.

Digoxin label. *Baxter Healthcare.*

Narcan, a medication used to increase respiration, is packaged in ampules. It is injected very slowly over 3 minutes. Once the desired parameter of respirations per minute is obtained, the drug is stopped.

What IS an Ampule?

An *ampule* is a sealed glass container that holds one dose of liquid or powdered medication. Ampules are not for multidose use. Examples of medications packaged in ampules include magnesium sulfate, diazepam (Valium), aminophylline, theophylline, and naloxone (Narcan).

Because ampules are made of glass, care must be taken when snapping them open.

Dispose of the rest of the vial and any unused medication in a hazard-proof box.

What You Need To KNOW

Ampules are often found in emergency code carts and in patient-medication draws. Because ampules are made of glass, you need to be careful when snapping them open.

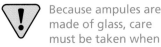
TAKE HOME POINTS

- Use a filter needle to withdraw the medication from an ampule, and change the needle before administering the medication to your patient.
- Do not attempt to get the rest of the medication out of the ampule by shaking it over a sink. Instead, place the ampule containing the unused medication into a hazard-proof box.
- Always snap the top of a vial away from your face to prevent the possibility of glass particles flying into your eyes.
- If available, use a filter needle to draw up medication from a vial to prevent aspiration of glass particles into the syringe.

What You DO

- Flick the top of the ampule with your index finger to move the liquid inside to the bottom.
- Get an alcohol wipe or 2 × 2 gauze pad, and wrap it around the top one third of the ampule. With a quick motion of the wrist, snap off the top of the ampule in a direction that is away from you.
- Discard the top of the ampule in a hazard-proof box.
- Obtain a filter needle, and draw up the desired amount of medication.

Do You UNDERSTAND?

DIRECTIONS: **Calculate the answers to the following questions.**

1. Mrs. Chebrianna is prescribed 2.5 mg diazepam (Valium) IM for mild anxiety. You have a 10-mL ampule with 5 mg/mL. How much Valium do you draw up into a syringe?_____

2. Jane Doe comes into the emergency department with a friend who says that Jane was "using lots of opioids tonight." Narcan is prescribed for acute opioid overdose at 0.8 mg IV now. You have 1-mL ampules of Narcan 0.4 mg/mL in stock. How many milliliters will you need to draw up into a syringe?_____

3. The prescription continues for Jane Doe. It states, "Narcan 0.2 mg every 2 to 3 minutes, until respirations reach 8 per minute." It has been 3 minutes, and Jane's respirations are at 5/min. How many milliliters of Narcan should you administer in the next dose?_____

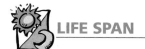

LIFE SPAN

Narcan is not recommended for neonates because it can cause cardiac irritability.

Pregnant women who require Narcan should be assessed for bleeding.

What IS a Transdermal Patch?

A *transdermal patch* is an adhesive, medicated disc that allows medication to be absorbed through the skin at a slow but relatively constant rate. Frequently used transdermal medications include nitroglycerin (NTG) patches, duragesic (fentanyl) patches, nicotine patches, and estrogen patches.

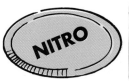

LIFE SPAN

Transdermal 17-beta-estradiol patch in nonobese, healthy postmenopausal women reduces the risk of developing type 2 diabetes.

TAKE HOME POINTS

Transdermal buprenorphine, an opioid analgesic, is effective in treating chronic pain by reducing pain intensity.

Transdermal therapeutic system: fentanyl (TTS-F) is effective in treating neuropathic pain.

What You NEED TO KNOW

Transdermal patches must be attached to hairless areas of skin that have not been irritated. If you need to remove hair before administering a transdermal patch, use scissors (not a razor) to prevent skin irritation. The upper chest, upper arms, and upper back are recommended sites for transdermal patch administration (you should avoid the use of distal areas of the extremities).

TAKE HOME POINTS

- Do not shave the area where you plan to place a transdermal patch. It can irritate the skin and adversely affect drug absorption.
- The rate of drug absorption with a transdermal patch varies according to skin condition, amount of physical exercise, and body temperature.
- Instruct your patients not to drink alcohol when on NTG. They could go into shock because of increased vasodilation.

Answers: 2. 2 mL; 3. 0.5 mL.

Duragesic Patches

- Conversion of oral morphine to duragesic patch is based on a 24-hour analgesic requirement.
- Confusion or hallucinations or both may occur within 72 hours of first applying a duragesic patch. These are not reasons to discontinue the medication. You should wait 72 hours until a blood level is established.
- The dose of a duragesic can be increased every 3 to 6 days, with the maximum dose being 300 mcg/hr for an adult. To prevent symptoms of abrupt narcotic withdrawal, discontinuation of a duragesic needs to be gradual.

Nitroglycerin Patches

- Discontinuation of NTG should be done over 4 to 6 weeks.
- NTG may stop preterm labor.
- Because a patient can develop a tolerance to NTG, the patch should be left on for 12 hours; then taken off for 12 hours (during sleep).
- To prevent explosion, NTG patches should be removed before defibrillation.

What You DO

- Assess your patient's level of pain on a 1 to 10 scale.
- Put on gloves and remove the previous patch.
- Be clear on the prescription. (To reduce the chance of the patient developing a tolerance to the drug, there may be an order for "12 hours on, 12 hours off.")
- Assess prescribed blood pressure (BP) and pulse parameters before applying the next patch. Usually the parameters indicate you should not apply the patch if an adult's systolic BP is less than 90 mm Hg or pulse is less than 60 beats/min.
- Wash the application area with water. (Avoid using creams, lotions, or soaps.)
- Let the area dry fully.
- Write the date, the time, and your initials on the patch.
- Remove the protective backing from the patch.
- Apply the patch to an irritation-free section of skin that is dry, fatty, and flat.

Assess prescribed BP and pulse parameters. You should not apply the patch if an adult's systolic BP less than 90 mm Hg or pulse is less than 60 beats/min.

- Hold the patch in place for 10 to 20 seconds to develop a seal.
- Tape over the patch to secure it in place, if desired.
- Remove your gloves.
- Chart the location of the patch.

Do You UNDERSTAND?

DIRECTIONS: **Answer the following questions.**

1. Mr. Samuels says his pain is a 9 on a scale of 1 to 10. He states, "I just can't take too much more of this pain." Mr. Samuels is currently receiving 50 mcg/hr of duragesic and has been at this dose for 1 week. You tell the prescribing professional that you feel his duragesic needs to be increased in strength. What new dose of duragesic would be best for Mr. Samuels?
   a. 25 mcg/hr
   b. 50 mcg/hr
   c. 75 mcg/hr
2. Because of her severe coronary artery disease, Mrs. Bernheart is suffering with angina pectoris. She is prescribed NTG 0.2 mg immediately during episodes of angina. This dose should be repeated every 5 minutes × 3. If she has no relief, she is to call the emergency squad (paramedics). What is the maximum total dose of NTG that Mrs. Bernheart could take before she calls the emergency squad?_____

What IS a Metered-Dose Inhaler?

A *metered-dose inhaler* (MDI) is a multidose aerosol device used for inhaling medications. Examples include albuterol sulfate (Proventil, Ventolin) and Combivent (ipratropium bromide plus albuterol sulfate). Steroid medications are often administered by MDI to treat long-term reactive airway disease.

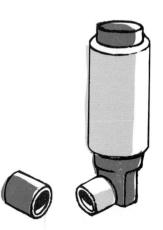

Answers: 1. c; 2. 0.8 mg.

What You NEED TO KNOW

Most MDIs are used to improve bronchodilation (i.e., breathing). The average adult dose to improve bronchodilation is two puffs every 4 to 6 hours for persons over 12 years old. Medications in inhalers can be self-administered by the patient by pressing down on the inhaler. If the patient is unable to do this manually, an adaptor can be used to provide mechanical ventilation.

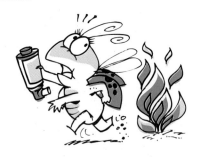

What You DO

You should assist or instruct your patient to do the following:
- Thoroughly shake the MDI.
- Test spray three times before using the inhaler if it is new or has not been used for several days.
- Rinse the mouth out with water.
- Inhale through the nose.
- Exhale through pursed lips or use diaphragmatic breathing to prolong expiration, and keep airways opened longer.
- Use a spacer, a tubelike device that ensures proper spacing between mouth and inhaler, or hold the inhaler two finger widths away before activating it.
- When pressing down on the inhaler, inhale completely and hold the inhalation for a minimum of 2 to 3 seconds (holding the inhalation for 10 seconds is preferred).
- Exhale through pursed lips.
- Inhale through the nose and exhale through pursed lips for 1 minute before beginning second puff (if prescribed).

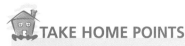

Do You UNDERSTAND?

1. If an inhaler is used only once a month, what is the procedure for test spraying?

   _____

2. Draw a mouth that shows the proper technique for self-administering a metered dose.

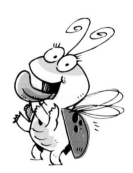

What IS a Sublingual Medication?

A *sublingual* (SL) *medication* is a small tablet or liquid medication that is placed under the tongue. Examples of sublingual medications include nifedipine (Procardia) to combat hypertension and NTG for angina pectoris.

> ⚠️ Procardia may increase the symptoms of angina when used in conjunction with beta-blocking medications.

What You NEED TO KNOW

- Some SL medications may sting or burn when placed under the tongue.
- NTG tablets are stored in brown-colored, light-resistant glass containers and must be discarded 6 months after opening.
- To decrease NTG's hypotensive effect, it is best to be lying down when taking the medication.
- If SL medications are placed in the buccal pouch instead of under the tongue, absorption of the medication will be slower.
- Store NTG in a cool, dry place with the cap of the bottle closed tightly.

🏠 TAKE HOME POINTS

- You should instruct your patients not to swallow SL medications, but to let them dissolve underneath their tongues.
- Because heat destroys the effectiveness of the medication, patients taking NTG should avoid storing it in their pockets or leaving it in a car.

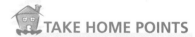

Answers: 1. **Test spray three times; 2. In the drawing, the mouth should be two finger widths away from the inhaler.**

What You DO

Assist or instruct your patients taking Procardia to do the following:
- Take the 10-mg capsule of Procardia and puncture a hole at one end of it with a sterile needle.
- Squeeze the contents of the capsule underneath the tongue.
- Monitor BP within 20 to 30 minutes for initial effect of the drug.

Assist or instruct your patients taking NTG to do the following:
- Place one tablet (gr $^1/_{150}$ to gr $^1/_{100}$ or 150 to 600 mcg) under the tongue and allow it to dissolve.
- Repeat with one tablet under the tongue every 5 minutes (for a total of three more tablets) if angina pain is not relieved.
- Spit out the remaining medication once pain is relieved to prevent the potential side effect of a headache.

TAKE HOME POINTS
- Your patients should not exceed a total of four NTG tablets for angina pain. (More than four tablets will decrease coronary blood flow by producing systemic hypotension.)
- If your patient experiences no relief after taking two NTG tablets, 911 should be called.

LIFE SPAN

Often older adults do not notice a burning or stinging sensation from the medication underneath their tongue.
Sublingual administration of allergen vaccines to children with asthma is a safe treatment and is known as sublingual immunotherapy (SLIT).

Do You UNDERSTAND?

DIRECTIONS: Answer the following questions.

1. Your patient has a history of angina pectoris and is prescribed Procardia for a hypertensive episode. What medications should you make sure the patient is not currently receiving to prevent increasing anginal symptoms?

   _____

2. Your 86-year-old grandmother has just taken NTG for chest pain. What position should her body be in to prevent hypotensive effects from the medication?

   _____

3. You have been asked to give a patient Procardia 20 mg SL now. You have 30 capsules in stock, each of which are 10 mg. How many capsules do you give the patient?

   _____

4. Which of the following is a normal dose of NTG? Place a check next to the correct answer.
   a. _____ 800 mcg
   b. _____ 50 mg
   c. _____ gr $^1/_{150}$
   d. _____ gr 25
   e. _____ 35 mEq

What IS an Enteral Medication?

An *enteral medication* is given by syringe, down a tube that goes into the stomach or intestines.

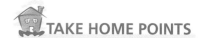
What You NEED TO KNOW

- Gastrostomy tube (G-tube) obstruction can result from superior mesenteric artery syndrome, a disorder in which the duodenum is compressed, resulting in delayed stomach emptying and medication absorption.
- Clamping a G-tube after instilling phenytoin medication increases the serum levels of phenytoin 1 hour after clamping.

What You DO

- Determine patency and correct placement of tube, if applicable.
- If a patient's G-tube appears to be partially obstructed (as evidenced by it being difficult to get liquid down the tube), try using a 5-mL or larger syringe to instill carbonated liquid (soda) or warm water into the tube. This should dissolve the clog.
- If unable to dissolve a clog in a G-tube, the tube must be discontinued by the prescribing professional.
- If no obstruction is present, determine the flow rate of solution, if necessary.
- Flush the tube with a minimum of 60 mL of water before and after each medication administration, unless this is contrary to the patient's plan of care.

 Never force liquid into a tube in an attempt to unclog it.

Do You UNDERSTAND?

DIRECTIONS: **Calculate the answers to the following questions.**

1. Mrs. Galloway is prescribed 10 mL of a multivitamin to be mixed with 230 mL of a nutritional supplement to run over 60 minutes. You have been asked to administer this prescription via a G-tube. The tubing used is 20 gtt/min. What should the flow rate be?

   _____

2. Mr. Inofeck is prescribed 20 mL of liquid Carafate (sucralfate) to be mixed in 80 mL of water to run over 15 minutes. The tubing used is 20 gtt/min. What should the flow rate be?

   _____

What IS a Prefilled-Syringe Medication?

A *prefilled-syringe medication* is a specific dose of a drug that has been prepackaged in a ready-to-use syringe. They are considered safe, convenient, and time saving. Examples include Lupron Depot form, meperidine hydrochloride (Demerol), sodium bicarbonate, $D_{50}W$, epinephrine autoinjector, and penicillin G.

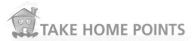

TAKE HOME POINTS

Replace any prefilled-syringe medications that have expired to prevent tragedy. For example, replacing outdated anaphylaxis medication kits will ensure that you are able to treat your patients for bee stings in an emergency.

What You NEED TO KNOW

- Each prefilled syringe is packaged with its own set of specific instructions and list of drug incompatibilities.
- A prefilled syringe can only be used once.

Answers: 1. 80 gtt/min; 2. 133.3 gtt/min (133 gtt/min when rounded down).

What You DO

When administering prefilled-syringe medications:
• Note the expiration date on the package.
• Determine that package is still sealed and that it contains all the necessary equipment.
• Administer the medication as prescribed in the package insert.
• Note any adverse reactions that your patient has to the medication, and report your findings to the prescribing professional.

Do You UNDERSTAND?

DIRECTIONS: **Answer the following questions.**

1. Lupron is an antineoplastic agent used for treating prostate cancer. The dose is 1 mg/day subcutaneously (SC), with a needle that is equal to or larger than a 22 gauge. Which needle should you use to administer Lupron?

   _____

2. Sodium bicarbonate, 200 to 300 mEq IV bolus, treats metabolic acidosis, which occurs during cardiopulmonary arrest. Sodium bicarbonate is not compatible with norepinephrine, dobutamine, or calcium-containing solutions. You are asked to give sodium bicarbonate to a patient who is in cardiac arrest. She has two IV lines running, one line with D_5W and one line with dobutamine. Which line should you use to administer the sodium bicarbonate?

   _____

3. Autoinjector epinephrine is used for treatment of anaphylaxis in children and adults who are allergic to bee stings. The dose is 0.3 mg for adults and 0.15 mg for children. You are doing your monthly assessment of medications in your family's home and determine that your daughter's autoinjector is out of date. What should you do?

   _____

Answers: 1. 18-gauge; 2. D_5W; 3. Discard the old autoinjector and obtain a new one immediately.

4. Mr. Holden comes into the emergency department with a blood sugar level of 44. He immediately is prescribed gr 25 of $D_{50}W$ IV. The label states $D_{50}W$, 1 gr = 2 mL $D_{50}W$. According to the label, how many milliliters of $D_{50}W$ should you give Mr. Holden?

References

Evans HC, Easthope SE: Transdermal buprenorphine, *Drugs* 63(19):1999-2012, 2003.

Lusardi P: Research corner. Do we need to filter medication ampules? Myth versus reality, *AACN News* 19(4):8, 2002.

Mattner F, Gastmeier P: Bacterial contamination of multidose vials: a prevalence study, *Am J Infect Control* 32(1):12-6, 2004.

Mystakidou K, Parpa E, Tsilika E et al: Long-term management of noncancer pain with transdermal therapeutic system—fentanyl, *J Pain* 4(6):298-306, 2003.

Pajno GB, Peroni DG, Vita D et al: Safety of sublingual immunotherapy in children with asthma, *Pediatr Drugs* 5(11):771-81, 2003.

Rossi R, Origliani G, Modena MG: Transdermal 17-s-estradiol and risk of developing type 2 diabetes in a population of healthy, nonobese postmenopausal women, *Diabetes Care* 27(3):645-9, 2004.

NCLEX® Review

Circle the correct answer.

1. Mr. Johnson is 85 years old and has been brought to the hospital emergency department with seizures of unknown cause. He is prescribed phenobarbital sodium 195 mg. You have a vial of phenobarbital sodium 130 mg/mL in stock. How much phenobarbital do you draw up in a syringe to give to Mr. Johnson?
   1 2 mL
   2 1.5 mL
   3 1 mL
   4 0.66 mL

2. A 32-year-old woman is brought into the emergency department in anaphylaxis because of a bee sting she received less than 3 minutes ago. You are asked to give 0.5 mg epinephrine SC immediately. The epinephrine comes in 30 mg vials at 1 mg/mL. How much epinephrine do you give the patient?
   1 60 mg
   2 2 mg
   3 0.2 mg
   4 0.5 mL

3. Mr. Hernendez is scheduled for surgery to remove a cyst in his abdomen. He is prescribed Demerol (meperidine hydrochloride) 100 mg, plus Vistaril (hydroxyzine) 25 mg IM immediately before surgery. You have a 20-mL multidose vial with Demerol 50 mg/mL and a 10-mL multidose vial with Vistaril 25 mg/mL. How many total milliliters should you draw up into one syringe when combining Demerol with Vistaril?
   1 3 mL
   2 4 mL
   3 6 mL
   4 10 mL

4. When using a metered-dose inhaler (MDI), the patient's mouth should be:
   1 Right on the inhaler
   2 Two finger widths away from the inhaler
   3 1 foot from the inhaler
   4 Within 6 inches of the inhaler

5. Mrs. Galloway is prescribed 5 mL of a multivitamin to be mixed with 85 mL of a nutritional supplement to run over 60 minutes. The tubing used is 20 gtt per minute. What should the flow rate be?
   1 4.5 gtt/min
   2 1.5 gtt/min
   3 13.33 gtt/min
   4 30 gtt/min

6. True or False? After adding a medication to an intravenous bag of fluid, you should invert the bag several times so the additive is distributed evenly.

7. Short answer: Anaphylaxis in a patient occurs following antibiotic treatment. The physician prescribes 1 mL of 1:1000 epinephrine subcutaneously. A multidose vial of epinephrine comes in 1:1000, 1 mg/mL. How much epinephrine do you draw up? _____

8. True or False? To open an ampule of medication, you use an alcohol wipe and snap off the top of the ampule in a direction that is towards your body.

9. Short answer: Your patient requires cardiac defibrillation and has a nitroglycerin medication patch on his chest. Why should you remove the nitroglycerin patch before defibrillation?

   _____

10. Short answer: When administering nitroglycerin intravenously you need to monitor what vital sign besides the pulse? _____

NCLEX® Review Answers

Notes

1. **2** 195:x = 130 : 1, so x = 1.5. If you answered 0.66 mL, you incorrectly reversed the two numbers that you divided.

2. **4** 0.5:x = 1:1, so x = 0.5. 60 mg is a lethal dose; you set up your proportion incorrectly.

3. **1** 100:x = 50:1 (Demerol), so x = 2 mL. Then 25:x = 1:1 (Vistaril), so x = 1. You add 2 + 1 = 3 mL.

4. **2** The patient's mouth should be two finger breadths to allow for maximum inhalation and maximum dose. The patient's mouth being placed directly on the inhaler inc reases inhalation resistance, and you loose the possibility of getting the maximum medication dose. Both 6 inches and 1 foot are too far away for inhalation.

5. **4** The flow rate is 30 gtt/min; you have used proportion and tubing rate correctly. If you answered 4.5 gtt/min, you did not set up the proportion correctly. If you answered 1.5 gtt/min, you forgot the tubing 20 gtt/min. If you answered 13.33 gtt/min, your ratio of 60/90 is incorrectly inverted.

6. True.

7. 1 mL.

8. False. Open in a direction away from your body to prevent glass getting in your eyes or face.

9. To prevent explosion and skin damage.

10. Blood pressure.

Medications
for Infants
and Children

What You WILL LEARN

After reading this chapter, you will know how to do the following:

✔ Name three common medications given to infants and/or children.

✔ Differentiate between types of medications and routes of administration for infants and children.

✔ Calculate dosages and methods of administration based on prescriptions for infants and children.

Administering medications to infants and children poses special challenges, including determining the correct drug doses for young patients. Infants are considered people ranging in age from birth to less than 24 months. Children are people ranging in age from 25 months to 150 months (12½ years) and weighing less than 150 lb.

What ARE Medications for Infants and Children?

Being able to calculate the correct *medication doses for infants and children* is essential to providing them with safe care. Because infants and children are smaller than most adults, they receive smaller doses of medication.

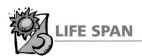

LIFE SPAN

Medication doses can be based on:
1. Age
2. Body surface area
3. Weight

Doses for younger patients are calculated based on their individual weight, age, or body surface area (BSA) (calculating doses based on BSA is the most accurate of these three methods).

What You NEED TO KNOW

Oral Medication Administration

Oral administration is the most preferred and least invasive method of giving medications to infants and children. Unless the infant or child cannot swallow oral medication or a particular drug is not effective in its oral form, medications should be given by this route. If administering medications orally is not an option, you should use nonoral delivery routes.

Because infants and children cannot swallow tablets easily (if at all), most oral drugs are prepared as liquids. Liquid medications for oral use are measured using a medication cup, a syringe, or a medication dropper calibrated in milliliters. You should shake liquid suspensions before pouring and measuring them because the active ingredient in a suspension tends to fall to the bottom of the bottle. Examples of liquid drug suspensions include the antibiotics amoxicillin plus potassium clavulanate (Augmentin), Septra (trimethoprim and sulfamethoxazole), and amoxicillin (Amoxil).

In some cases, you will need to administer tablets and capsules to children (you will never administer tablets or capsules to infants). After giving the child the medication, you must check the oral cavity (i.e., mouth) to make sure that the medication has been completely swallowed. Keep in mind that a common trick among younger patients is to hide the tablet or capsule under their tongues so that they can spit it out when health care providers are not looking. Therefore be sure to instruct young patients to lift up their tongues when making the inspection after swallowing.

To disguise bad-tasting drugs and encourage young patients to take medications, some tablets or capsules can be crushed and placed in a small amount of applesauce or ice cream.

Intramuscular Medication Administration

Some drugs must be administered to infants and children intramuscularly (IM) because of their absorption properties or because they are only

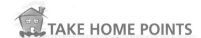

TAKE HOME POINTS

- Do not mix bad-tasting medications with a child's favorite food. (This could create an association between a bad or "funny" taste and the food, and prevent the child from eating it in the future.)
- Do not crush time-released or enteric-coated medications.

manufactured as IM medications. Because the gluteal muscles do not develop until children learn to walk, the best IM injection sites for infants and children are the vastus lateralis or rectus femoris muscles of the thigh.

Common IM medications include those used preoperatively and postoperatively for sedation or pain control, and immunizations for diphtheria, pertussis, and tetanus (DPT) and measles, mumps, and rubella (MMR).

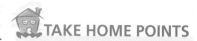
TAKE HOME POINTS

Most medications have no effect on milk supply or infant well-being but always consult reliable sources. Fluoxetine (Prozac) should be avoided in breast-feeding women.

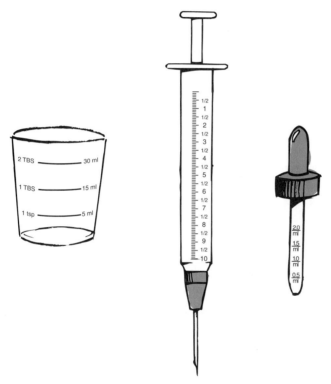

Intravenous Medication Administration

Because infants and children have small muscle size, many drugs are administered intravenously (IV) rather than IM. The veins of your young patients are extremely fragile, so you must carefully examine any potential IV site and choose the correct catheter size before administering the medication. Many IV medications are given within a 24-hour period (e.g., antibiotics are usually administered over 30 to 60 minutes and involve several doses within a 24-hour period). Other IV medications, such as aminophylline for bronchodilation, are administered to the patient over several hours.

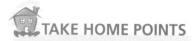
TAKE HOME POINTS

IV infusion in infants for longer periods of time are usually given through either a central line, veins in the temporal region of the scalp, or at times in the back of the hand or dorsum of the foot.

What You DO

Five general principles should be remembered when giving medications to infants or children:

1. Determine the medication or medications to be given.
2. Determine the least invasive way of administering the drug or drugs.
3. Calculate the proper dose or doses to be administered.
4. Administer the medication or medications.
5. Evaluate the effectiveness and side effects of the medication or medications.

Oral and Intramuscular Medication Calculations

Several mathematical formulas are used to determine medication doses for infants and children. Although nomograms are used to estimate BSA based on height and weight of the child (see Chapter 2, "Systems of Measurement"), you can also use the following formulas to calculate medication doses based on your patient's BSA:

$$\text{Infant or child's dose} = (\text{surface area}/1.7 \text{ m}^2) \times \text{normal adult dose}$$

OR

$$\frac{\text{BSA of child (m}^2)}{\text{BSA of adult } (1.7 \times \text{m}^2)} \times \text{normal adult dose}$$

You can also use the following formula to calculate oral and IM doses for your young patients based only on their weight:

$$\text{mg of medication} \times \text{weight in kilograms (mg/kg)}$$

Although you can use the same calculation methods to determine oral and IM medication doses, you should always measure IM medications to the nearest hundredth.

Intravenous Medication Calculation

Because infants can only tolerate a narrow range of hydration, you must take great care in assessing drug doses, drug dilutions, and the associated flow rate when administering IV medications to your youngest patients. Remember that all IV medications given to infants and children should be administered with an electric pump or controller, such as a Buretrol.

Do NOT administer more than 1 mL per IM site to prevent absorption disruption and tissue damage.

You can use the following formulas to calculate the flow rate of IV medications:

$$\text{flow rate in gtt/min (drops/minute)}$$
$$= (\text{total volume} \times \text{set calibration}) \div \text{time in minutes}$$

OR

$$\text{volume} \times \text{calibration time in hours} = \text{milliliters/hour}$$

Sites for IM Injections in Infants and Children

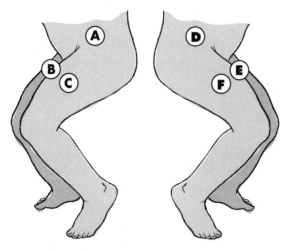

When administering an IV medication over several hours, you should inject the correct amount of medication into a mini-IV bag or a small, round, precise measuring tube (calibrated burette) that is connected to the IV line. For IV medications administered in several doses over a 24-hour period, you should use a calibrated burette. After administering the medication to children, you should follow with 15 mL of flush for peripheral lines and 20 mL of flush for central lines. For infants, 5 mL of flush is used for peripheral lines and 10 mL for central lines.

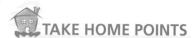

TAKE HOME POINTS

In addition to calculating safe doses, you must understand drug actions, side effects, and signs of toxicity.

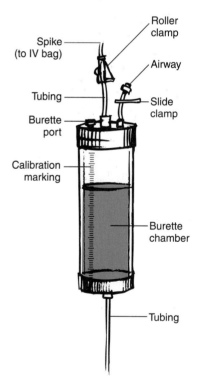

Roller clamp
Spike (to IV bag)
Airway
Tubing
Slide clamp
Burette port
Calibration marking
Burette chamber
Tubing

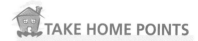

TAKE HOME POINTS

A burette holds 100 to 150 mL, and it is calibrated in 1 mL increments.

Do You UNDERSTAND?

DIRECTIONS: Prepare the following doses of oral medications for a young patient based on the available dose and prescription. Note that neither weight, age, nor BSA are necessary to complete these exercises.

1. Amoxicillin/clavulanate potassium (Augmentin). Available dose 125 mg/5 mL. The prescription reads 125 mg twice daily (BID). Patient dose = _____ mL Augmentin.
2. Digoxin (Lanoxin) elixir. Available dose = 0.05 mg/cc. The prescription reads 0.1 mg. Patient dose = _____ cc Lanoxin.
3. Acetaminophen (Tylenol). Available dose = 60 mg/0.5 mL. The prescription reads 120 mg. Patient dose = _____ mL acetaminophen.
4. Erythromycin. Available dose = 200 mg/5 mL. The prescription reads 300 mg now. Patient dose = _____ mL erythromycin.

DIRECTIONS: Calculate the appropriate doses for a young patient based on weight in kilograms (weight in pounds divided by 2.2 equals weight in kilograms, or 1 lb ÷ 2.2 = 1 kg).

5. A 3-year-old child who weighs 14 kg. The recommended dose of meperidine (Demerol) for a child is 1.1 mg/kg/dose. Child's dose = _____.
6. A 4-year-old child who weighs 18 kg. The recommended dose of gentamicin sulfate (Garamycin) for a child is 7.5 mg/kg/day. Child dose every 6 hours = _____.
7. A 3-month-old infant who weighs 4 kg. The recommended dose of morphine for an infant is 0.1 mg/kg/dose. Infant dose = _____.
8. An 8-year-old child who weighs 64 lb. The recommended dose of aspirin is 65 mg/kg/day. Child dose every 4 hours = _____.
9. A 6-year-old child who weighs 50 lb. The recommended dose of clindamycin is 25 mg/kg/day. Child dose every 8 hours = _____.

Answers: 1. 5 mL; 2. 2 cc; 3. 1 mL; 4. 7.5 mL; 5. 15.4 mg/dose; 6. 33.75 mg q6h; 7. 0.4 mg/dose; 8. 314 mg; 9. 189 mg q8h.

DIRECTIONS: **Use BSA to calculate the appropriate doses.**

10. An adult dose of phenobarbital is 5 mg/kg/day. The patient weighs 7 kg, and BSA = 1.31m². What is the total daily dose of phenobarbital?

_____

11. An adult dose of ampicillin is 200 mg/kg/day. The patient weighs 12 kg, and BSA = 0.51m². What is the total daily dose of ampicillin?

_____

DIRECTIONS: **Prepare the following IM medications.**

12. Meperidine (Demerol) for pain relief. The available dose = 25 mg/mL, and the prescription reads 20 mg. Patient dose = _____ mL Demerol.

13. Atropine for preoperative administration. The available dose = 0.4 mg/mL, and the prescription reads 0.1 mg. Patient dose = _____ mL atropine.

14. Morphine for postoperative pain. The available dose = 15 mg/mL, and the prescription reads 10 mg. Patient dose = _____ _____ mL morphine.

15. Connect the words appropriate for peripheral administration of an antibiotic to a child over a 24-hour period. What word abbreviation does it spell?

24 hr	oral	rate	infant	flush
burette	SQ	teaspoon	volume	artery

16. What is the flow rate in drops per minute if:
    Volume = 10 mL
    Flush = 15 mL
    Set calibration = 60 gtt/mL
    Time = 20 minutes
    Flow rate = _____ gtt/min.

17. The prescription is for an antibiotic, vancomycin hydrochloride (Vancocin), 250 mg in 5 mL, to be diluted for a total of 40 mL volume and infused over 60 minutes. The set calibration is 60 gtt/min, and a 15 mL flush follows. What is the flow rate in drops per minute? Flow rate = _____ gtt/min.

References

Della-Giustina K, Chow G. Medications in pregnancy and lactation, *Emerg Med Clin N Am* 21(3): 585-613, 2003.

Digman J: *Pediatric medication administration,* Irvine, Calif, 1998, Concept Media.

Gjerdingen D. The effectiveness of various postpartum depression treatments and the impact of antidepressant drugs on nursing infants, *J Am Board Fam Pract* 16(5):372-82, 2003.

NCLEX® Review

Circle the correct answer.

1. An infant is defined as a person who is less than how many months old?
   1 6
   2 12
   3 24
   4 36

2. With infants, most parenteral medications are given by the IV route (as opposed to the IM route) because infants have:
   1 Little subcutaneous fat
   2 A hard time swallowing
   3 A large BSA
   4 Small muscle size

3. A 6-month-old infant weighing 5 kg is prescribed 1 mg of morphine before surgery for a diagnostic test. The recommended dose of morphine for an infant is 0.1 mg/kg/dose. Is the prescribed dose of morphine safe or unsafe?
   1 Safe
   2 Unsafe

4. Which of the following medications should you not crush?
   1 Enteric-coated aspirin tablet
   2 Acetaminophen (Tylenol) tablet
   3 Phenobarbital tablet
   4 Cimetidine (Tagamet) tablet

5. Which of the following medications needs to be shaken before pouring the required dose?
   1 Docusate sodium (Colace) liquid
   2 Acetaminophen (Tylenol) gel cap
   3 Cefaclor (Ceclor) liquid suspension
   4 Isosorbide dinitrate sustained-release capsule

6. True or False? Body surface area is the most accurate method for determining doses of medications for infants and children.

7. True or False? Liquid medications for oral use are calibrated in milliliters.

8. Fill in the blank: You should _____ liquid suspensions of medications before pouring them because the active ingredient in the suspension tends to fall to the bottom of the bottle.

9. Short answer: Why are the gluteal muscles not good sites for intramuscular injections in infants? _____
   _____

10. Short answer: What is the maximum amount, in milliliters, per site that should be administered in an intramuscular injection for a child?
    _____

NCLEX® Review Answers

1. **3** An infant is younger than 24 months, which is considered the infant stage because medications are still given within the weight range classified for infants and physical development is younger than that of a child. At 36 months of age, the weight range is within that of children and more physically that of an adult.

2. **4** Infant muscles are small, but this is in proportion to their small body size. Infants have more subcutaneous fat. Most infants have no problems swallowing and have a small BSA.

3. **2** It is unsafe because 0.1 mg × 5 kg = 0.5 mg/dose.

243

4. **1** Enteric-coated medications should not be crushed. Acetaminophen, phenobarbital, and cimetidine tablets are not enterically coated.

5. **3** Suspensions need to be shaken because they are medications mixed with another substance. Liquids and capsules do not need to be shaken.

6. True.

7. True.

8. shake.

9. The gluteal muscles are not developed in infants because they are not walking yet; hence drug absorption would be affected.

10. 1 mL.

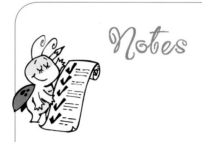

Notes

Advanced Care

What You WILL LEARN

After reading this chapter, you will know how to do the following:

- ✔ Recognize and select appropriate specialty medications such as dopamine, nipride, dobutamine, vasopressin, heparin sodium, intravenous nitroglycerin, and vitamin K.
- ✔ Read and interpret patient prescriptions of specialty medications.
- ✔ Calculate rates and determine method of administration of specialty medications based on prescription and patient's clinical condition.

Providing care for patients who are critically ill requires advanced knowledge of certain medications and their doses. Some of the most common medications given in advanced-care settings include dopamine, nitroprusside, dobutamine, vasopressin, heparin sodium, nitroglycerin (NTG), and vitamin K. Most of these drugs are given intravenously (IV), either by flow rate (milliliters/hour or drops/minute) or by dose (mcg/kg/min, mcg/kg/hr, or Units/kg/min), and the rate of administration is adjusted, or titrated, according to set parameters.

Because this chapter covers advanced concepts, you may find it too complex. If you do, you may want to skim it, then reread it, and complete the "Do You UNDERSTAND?" questions when you study critical care or advanced medical-surgical nursing.

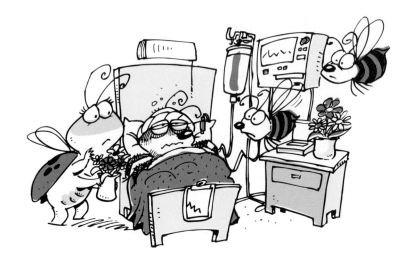

What IS Dopamine?

Dopamine (Intropin, Dopastat, Revimine) is an IV injectable medication that produces effects associated with the stimulation of the sympathetic nervous system (sympathomimetic agent). Dopamine causes renal, mesenteric, and cerebral artery vasodilation (i.e., a dopaminergic effect) in drug dosages less than 3 mcg/kg/min. In moderate dosages, between 3 and 10 mcg/kg/min, it improves blood pressure (BP) in nonhypovolemic states of shock. In higher dosages (above 10 mcg/kg/min), dopamine causes the release of norepinephrine and stimulates alpha receptors.

There are two main reasons that you need to monitor patients receiving dopamine:

1. Sudden increases in BP can cause cerebrovascular accidents (CVA) in the brain, myocardial infarction (MI) of the heart, increased oozing of surgical and bone marrow aspiration sites, oozing of vascular suture lines, and aortic aneurysm oozing.

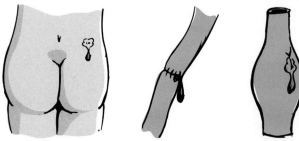

2. Peripheral vasoconstriction can cause blood to move slowly (stasis) to the extremities and increase vascular thrombosis and tissue ischemia, especially in persons with peripheral vascular disease (PVD) or diabetes mellitus (DM).

Dopamine is used to treat congestive heart failure (CHF), hypertension, occlusive vascular disease, and early renal insufficiency. The actions of dopamine are listed in the following table.

Actions of Dopamine

Dosage	Physiology	Effect
Low = 1 to 3 mcg/kg/min	Renal vasodilation	⇑ Renal blood flow ⇑ Urine output ⇑ Sodium excretion
Moderate = 3 to 10 mcg/kg/min	⇑ Norepinephrine release	⇑ Heart contractility ⇑ Cardiac stroke volume ⇑ Cardiac output
High = 11 to 50 mcg/kg/min	Stimulates alpha receptors	⇑ Peripheral vascular resistance ⇑ Systolic and diastolic BP

What You NEED TO KNOW

- Dopamine's onset is 1 to 5 minutes, with a duration of 10 minutes.
- The patient's weight must be determined to calculate correctly the dose of medication required.
- After administering dopamine, patients should be continuously monitored for baseline BP, cardiac rate and respirations, and vital signs every 15 minutes.
- The dose is carefully increased (titrated up) as prescribed.
- You must remember to assess the patient's BP before increasing the dose.
- Determine (with the prescribing professional) the parameters for adjusting the rate of dopamine and the steps for discontinuing infusion.
- To prevent hypotension, dopamine doses should be decreased (tapered down) before they are discontinued.

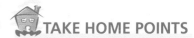
TAKE HOME POINTS

In most cases, dopamine is not prescribed for patients who have pulmonary edema. Vasoconstrictive effects of the drug increase venous return and pulmonary blood flow, resulting in increased ventricular pressure. This can worsen the pulmonary edema.

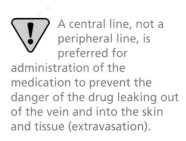
A central line, not a peripheral line, is preferred for administration of the medication to prevent the danger of the drug leaking out of the vein and into the skin and tissue (extravasation).

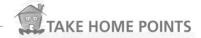
TAKE HOME POINTS

Doses of dopamine come in 40, 80, and 160 mg/mL ampules (to be diluted).
Flow rates include milliliters/hr and drops/minute.
Conversion to memorize is 1000 mcg = 1 mg.

Three steps can be used to calculate the dose of dopamine from the flow rate:

Step 1: Determine the dose per hour.

Step 2: Convert milligrams to micrograms.

Step 3: Convert micrograms/hour to micrograms/minute.

EXAMPLE: **You have 500 mL D$_5$W to which you add 400 mg of dopamine. This is to infuse at 400 mcg/min IV. What is the flow rate?**

Step 1: 400 mcg/min × 60 min = 24,000 mcg/hr

Step 2: 24,000 mcg/hr = 24 mg/hr

Step 3: 400 mg : 500 mL = 24 mg : x mL

   Answer: x = 30 mL/hr (gtt/min)

EXAMPLE: **You have 500 mL D$_5$W plus 800 mg dopamine at 25 mL/hr IV. What is the dose?**

Step 1: 800 mg : 500 mL = x mg : 25 mL; x = 40 mg/hr

Step 2: 40 mg/hr = 40,000 mcg/hr

Step 3: 40,000 mcg/hr 60 min =666.6

   Answer: 667 mcg/min (rounded up from 666.6)

Four steps can be used to calculate the flow rate from the dose of dopamine per kilogram of patient weight:

Step 1: Calculate the dose per minute.

Step 2: Calculate the dose per hour.

Step 3: Convert to like units.

Step 4: Calculate milliliters per hour flow rate.

EXAMPLE: **You have dopamine presecribed at 10 mcg/kg/min. You have a 250 mL bag of D$_5$W with 400 mg of dopamine in it, and the patient weighs 80 kg. What is the flow rate?**

Step 1: 80 kg × mcg/min = 800 mcg/min

Step 2: 800 mcg/min × 60 min = 48,000 mcg/hr

Step 3: 48,000 mcg = 48 mg/hr

Step 4: 400 mg : 250 mL = 48 mg : x mL

   Answer: x = 30 mL/hr (gtt/min)

Four steps can be used to determine the desired dose of dopamine in milliliters per hour:

Step 1: Multiply the drug prescribed of mcg/kg/min by the patient's weight in kilograms.

Step 2: Multiply this number by 60 (this gives you the microgram dose per hour).

Step 3: Divide the microgram dose per hour by 1000 to obtain milligrams per hour.

Step 4: Multiply this number by concentration of milliliters per milligram to equal milliliters per hour.

EXAMPLE: **You have 6 mcg/kg/min of dopamine, and the patient weighs 198 lb. Your concentration is 800 mg/500 mL. What is the milliliter per hour rate of dopamine?**

Step 1: 198 lb 2.2 = 90 kg in weight, so 6 mcg/kg/min × 90 = 540 mcg/min

Step 2: 540 × 60 = 32,400 mcg/hr

Step 3: 32,400 divided by 1000 = 32.4 mg/hr

Step 4: 32.4 mg/hr × 500 mL/800 mg = 20.25 mL/hr

Answer: The desired dose of dopamine is 20.25 mL/hr.

What You DO

- Determine cardiac output and pulmonary-wedge pressure according to facility policy—usually every 2 hours but at least once a shift.
- Assess peripheral pulses, color and temperature of extremities, and urinary output every 30 minutes.
- Assess for signs of excessive vasoconstriction (e.g., decreased urine output, tachycardia or dysrhythmia, decreased pulse pressure, cool extremities, and delayed capillary refill [greater than 3 seconds indicates a problem]).
- Reduce the dose of dopamine to $\frac{1}{10}$ the calculated amount for patients currently taking monoamine oxidase (MAO) inhibitor medications or who have taken them within the last 3 weeks.
- If IV extravasation of dopamine occurs, stop the infusion immediately and infiltrate the area intradermally with 10 to 15 mL of 0.9% sodium chloride (NaCl) solution containing 5 to 10 mg of phentolamine mesylate.

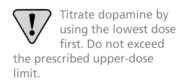

Titrate dopamine by using the lowest dose first. Do not exceed the prescribed upper-dose limit.

Do You UNDERSTAND?

DIRECTIONS: **Use calculations to find the answers.**

1. Each ampule of dopamine contains 80 mg/mL. You are asked to add 5 ampules to 500 mL D$_5$W and infuse at 25 mL/hr. What is the correct calculation?

2. The prescription on a patient care map reads, "Dopamine 5 mcg/kg/min." The solution is 250 mL D$_5$W, with 400 mg of dopamine added, and your patient weighs 70 kg. What flow rate should you program into the electronic-monitoring device attached to the patient's IV?

3. The prescription for your patient reads, "500 mL D$_5$NS. Add 600 mg dopamine, and infuse at 200 mcg/min IV." What is the milliliter per hour rate?

4. The prescription for your patient reads, "5 mcg/kg/min of dopamine." The patient weighs 142 lb, and your concentration of dopamine is 800 mg/500 mL. What is the rate in milliliter per hour?

What IS Nipride?

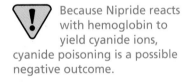

Because Nipride reacts with hemoglobin to yield cyanide ions, cyanide poisoning is a possible negative outcome.

Nipride (e.g., nitropress and nitroprusside sodium) is a vasodilator of the arterioles and venous smooth muscles that decreases peripheral vascular resistance and increases cardiac output. When Nipride is used, a patient's cardiac output increases because of a decrease in preload (PCWP) and afterload (SVR). This medication is used to treat hypertension, to treat CHF (in combination with dopamine), and to reduce bleeding after surgery.

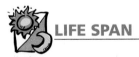

LIFE SPAN

Average adult IV infusion of Nipride is 3 mcg/kg/min. Average pediatric IV infusion of Nipride is 1.4 mcg/kg/min.

What You NEED TO KNOW

- Once an IV solution is mixed with Nipride, the solution is only good for 24 hours.
- Reconstitution of each vial, with 2 to 3 mL of 5% dextrose or sterile water, is required before injecting Nipride into an IV bag.
- If Nipride leaks into surrounding tissues, it will produce extreme pain and tissue sloughing.
- Rapid infusion of Nipride causes severe hypotension. Symptoms such as nausea, vomiting, headache, sweating, restlessness, dizziness, and heart palpitations are possible.
- Therapeutic response to Nipride should be seen within 2 to 5 minutes (10 minutes maximum) of drug infusion.
- If no response is seen to Nipride after 10 minutes, the medication should be discontinued by titrating down the IV.

    Four steps can be used to calculate the flow rate per kilogram of Nipride:

    Step 1: Calculate the dose per minute.
    Step 2: Determine the dose per hour.
    Step 3: Convert to like units.
    Step 4: Determine the milliliter per hour flow rate.

> ⚠ In some cases Nipride can cause cardiac dysrhythmia.

EXAMPLE: **Infuse Nipride, 50 mg in 500 mL D$_5$W at 2 mcg/kg/min, for a patient who weighs 58 kg.**

    Step 1: 58 kg × 2 mcg/min = 116 mcg/min
    Step 2: 116 mcg/min × 60 min = 6960 mcg/hr
    Step 3: 6960 mcg = 6.96 mg = 7 mg/hr
    Step 4: 50 mg : 500 mL = 7 mg : x mL, with x = 70 mL/hr

    Answer: The flow rate should be set at 70 mL/hr, which equals 70 gtt/min.

What You DO

- Look at the bag of fluid containing Nipride to be sure the solution is not deteriorated.
- Make sure the bag is labeled with a 24-hour sticker.

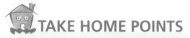

If the solution is deteriorated, do not use it. Good solution is a faint brown color, whereas deteriorated solution includes the colors of blue, green, or dark red.

TAKE HOME POINTS

- Rate of infusion should not exceed 10 mcg/kg/hr.
- Nipride is only compatible with D$_5$W.

- Dilute prepared Nipride into 250 to 1000 mL of D$_5$W for a concentration of 50 mcg/mL. (Normally you will use 250 mL or 500 mL bags of D$_5$W for dilution.)
- Protect the bag from light by covering it.
- Provide continuous electrocardiographic (ECG) and BP monitoring for patients receiving Nipride.
- Assess your patients for signs of metabolic acidosis (e.g., weakness, disorientation, headache, nausea, vomiting, and hyperventilation).
- Assess your patients for signs of cyanide toxicity (e.g., blurred vision, tinnitus, confusion, hyperreflexia, and seizures).
- Nipride is only compatible with D$_5$W.

Do You UNDERSTAND?

DIRECTIONS: Use calculations to find the answers.

1. A 58-year-old man who weighs 70 kg complains of severe chest pain. Nipride is prescribed as follows: Nipride 50 mg in 500 mL D$_5$W at 2 mcg/kg/min. What is the flow rate in milliliters/hour (drops/minute)?

2. A 72-year-old woman is scheduled to receive Nipride, which can be titrated from 3 to 6 mcg/kg/min. The solution is 50 mg Nipride in 250 mL D$_5$W, and your patient weighs 72 kg. What is the flow rate in milliliters per hour for the lower dose of 3 mcg/kg/min? What is the flow rate in milliliters per hour for the upper dosage of 6 mcg/kg/min?

What IS Dobutamine?

Dobutamine hydrochloride (Dobutrex) is a synthetic sympathomimetic that increases cardiac output while only mildly increasing heart rate and BP. The net effects of this medication are similar to the effects produced by a combination of dopamine and Nipride. However, this drug has a lower incidence of producing heart dysrhythmia. Dobutamine is used to treat patients who have pulmonary edema, low cardiac output, low BP, heart failure after cardiac surgery, or a right ventricular MI.

What You NEED TO KNOW

- When administering dobutamine to a patient, remember that the onset of drug action is 1 to 2 minutes, and that plasma half-life is 2 minutes.
- Because dobutamine is metabolized in the liver, good liver function is necessary.
- Usually BP in patients receiving dobutamine increases 10 to 20 mm Hg, and heart rate increases 5 to 15 beats/min.
- Reconstitution of the drug is done using normal saline (NS) or D_5W. (After mixing, oxidation may cause a slight color change. However, drug potency is not affected.)
- You must remember that drug-to-drug interactions can occur with dobutamine. (For example, dobutamine interacts with β-adrenergic blocking agents [e.g., propranolol], MAO inhibitors, antidepressants, nitroprusside, and general anesthetics [e.g., halothane and cyclopropane].)

 Dobutamine is incompatible with sodium bicarbonate solution.

What You DO

- Continuously assess your patient's BP and ECG output during drug administration.
- Assess the patient's cardiac output and pulmonary artery wedge pressure (PAWP) using a Swan-Ganz catheter before and within 2 minutes after drug administration.
- Infuse at a rate of 2 to 10 mcg/kg/min as prescribed.
- Assess your patients for signs of adverse reaction, such as nausea, vomiting, shortness of breath (SOB), headache, paresthesia, leg cramps, fatigue, nervousness, preventricular contractions (PVCs) on the ECG, and anginal pain.
- Monitor the patient's intake and output hourly.

Do You UNDERSTAND?

DIRECTIONS: Use calculations to find the answer.

1. Mr. Rollenbin has a low cardiac output with mild hypertension. He is prescribed dobutamine 50 mg in 500 mL D_5W at 2 mcg/kg/min. He weighs 58 kg. How many drops per minute (drops/minute) of the dobutamine solution should he receive?

   _____

DIRECTIONS: Fill in the blanks.

2. The major advantage of dobutamine is that it increases cardiac output while only mildly increasing two vital signs: _____ and _____.

3. For the metabolism of dobutamine to occur, the _____ needs to be in good working order?

What IS Vasopressin?

Vasopressin (Pitressin, Pressyn), a hormone secreted by the hypothalamus, can be given as a medication by several routes: into the nose, into an artery, intramuscularly (IM), subcutaneously (SC), or IV. This drug is used to prevent excessive urination (polyuria) in persons with diabetes insipidus (see box following). It is also used to treat postoperative abdominal distention, intestinal paresis, and acute massive hemorrhage (e.g., esophageal varices, acute gastritis, and brain hemorrhage). Medications that interfere with vasopressin include ethanol, reserpine, morphine sulfate, phenytoin, and chlorpromazine.

Vasopressin works in three ways: (1) it increases reabsorption of water through the renal tubules (this decreases urinary flow), (2) it stimulates the contraction of smooth muscles (this prevents abdominal distention and intestinal standstill), and (3) it causes vasoconstriction (this causes reduced blood flow to the heart, brain, lungs, bowel, and peripheral body areas).

Answers: 1. 70 gtt/min (58 kg × 3 mcg/min = 116 mcg/min. 116 mcg/min × 60 minutes = 6960 mcg/hr. 6960 mcg/hr ÷ 1000 mg = 6.96 mg = 7 mg/hr. Your proportion becomes 50 mg : 500 mL = 7 mg : x mL. x = 70 mL/hr = 70 gtt/min); 2. heart rate and BP; 3. liver.

Causes of Diabetes Insipidus

Encephalitis	Renal disease, advanced
Polycystic kidney disease	Meningitis
Head trauma	Sarcoidosis
Pregnancy	Metastatic breast cancer
Hypothalamus tumor	Syphilis
Pyelonephritis	Pituitary tumor
Medullary cystic disease	Tuberculosis

What You NEED TO KNOW

- The duration of vasopressin is 30 minutes to 1 hour IV, and 2 to 8 hours IM or SC.
- Because vasopressin is excreted in the urine, side effects (e.g., stomach cramps, nausea, vomiting, and skin blanching) can be reduced by giving the patient one to two glasses of water at the time of IM or SC administration.
- Vasopressin doses differ by route, age, and condition (see following table).
- Combining vasopressin with NTG or Nipride reduces the unwanted cardiac side effects (e.g., decreased coronary blood flow and decreased cardiac contractility) produced by vasopressin alone.

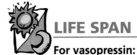

LIFE SPAN

For vasopressin:
Assess older patients for signs of water intoxication (e.g., drowsiness, headache, and listlessness).
   Monitor older patients for signs of MI (caused by toxic effects of the drug).

Vasopressin Administration

Condition	Route	Age
Diabetes insipidus	IM, SC	Adults = 5 to 15 Units bid or qid Older adults = 5 to 10 Units bid or qid Children = 2.5 to 10 Units bid or qid
Abdominal distention	IM	Adults = 5 to 10 Units q3h to q4h
Gastrointestinal hemorrhage	IV Intraarterial	Adults and older adults = 0.2 to 0.9 Units/min

What You DO

- Obtain a history of the patient's hypersensitivity or anaphylaxis to vasopressin to use as a baseline. This history should include the patient's weight, BP, pulse, and results of serum electrolytes and urine specific gravity.
- If administering vasopressin by IM or SC routes, give the patient one to two glasses of water to decrease gastrointestinal side effects.
- IV vasopressin can be mixed with D_5W or NS to concentrations of 0.1 to 1 Units/mL.
- Monitor intake and output (e.g., ECG output, level of consciousness, lung sounds, and daily weight).
- Evaluate injection site for pain, erythema, and abscess formation.
- Discontinue vasopressin if chest pain or anaphylaxis occurs.
- Report symptoms of headache and/or SOB to the prescribing professional immediately.

Do You UNDERSTAND?

DIRECTIONS: Provide the correct answers.

1. List the five routes by which vasopressin can be administered.

   _____

   _____

   _____

   _____

   _____

DIRECTIONS: Fill in the correct arrow.

2. Vasopressin increases reabsorption of water through the renal tubules. This means that urinary output in the patient receiving vasopressin will be:

a

b

DIRECTIONS: **Provide the correct answers.**

3. What two nursing interventions should you be aware of before giving vasopressin by the IM route?

a. _____

b. _____

DIRECTIONS: **Check the correct answer.**

4. Your patient begins an infusion of vasopressin as prescribed. He motions to you that he is having difficulty breathing. He also has an increased temperature and hives on his chest. Your *first* nursing interventions should be to:

a. _____ Notify the physician

b. _____ Obtain the crash cart

c. _____ Administer antidiuretic hormone IV

d. _____ Discontinue vasopressin

e. _____ Give two glasses of water to the patient

f. _____ Give 1:1000 solution of epinephrine SC

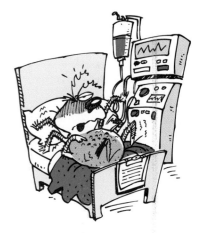

What IS Heparin Sodium?

Heparin sodium (e.g., Liquaemin and Hepalean) is an anticoagulant medication that slows the growth of existing blood clots and inhibits new clot formations. Doses of this medication are calculated on an individual basis according to the results of activated partial thromboplastin time (APTT) blood tests. Heparin sodium is used to treat deep vein thrombosis (DVT), pulmonary embolism, unstable angina, and atrial fibrillation. It is also administered to patients recovering from an MI, angioplasty, or prosthetic heart valve replacement (to prevent reclotting).

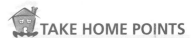

TAKE HOME POINTS

Heparin sodium does not dissolve blood clots; it only slows their growth and formation.

What You NEED TO KNOW

- A normal adult dose of heparin is 20,000 to 40,000 Units (USP units) q24h.
- A common starting dose for heparin in a patient with a DVT is 5000 Units of heparin bolus, followed by an infusion of 1000 Units/hr. Adjustment of the rate and dose follows after the APTT results are obtained.
- When the concentration is known, heparin is prescribed in either units per hour or milliliters per hour, and the dose can be based on the patient's weight (see box following).
- The half-life of heparin is less than 1 hour.
- Use of NTG reduces heparin's effectiveness.
- Standard weight-based doses include a bolus of 80 Units/kg and infusion of 18 Units/kg/hr.
- The therapeutic range of the laboratory value of APTT for thrombo-embolitic disease is 1.5 to 2.5 times the laboratory control value. (Range depends on the reagent used to run the APTT test, so check with your laboratory personnel.)
- To counteract the effect of heparin sodium, patients are given protamine sulfate. For IV heparin administration, 25 to 50 mg of protamine sulfate is used; for intermittent subcutaneous heparin dosing, 1.0 to 1.5 mg of protamine sulfate for every 100 Units heparin is given.

Advantages of Heparin Sodium

- Therapeutic level of anticoagulation is reached sooner—within 8 hours—compared with 24 hours when weight not used.
- Administration is safe and has fewer bleeding complications.
- Rate of recurrence of DVT is decreased.
- Hospital stay is decreased, and the chance of readmission is reduced.

What You DO

- Weigh the patient daily for weight-based heparin dosing.
- Make sure APTT is drawn q6h in critical care patients (or as prescribed) so that heparin dosing adjustments can be made.

- Noncritical care patients usually have APTTs drawn daily; then weekly for 1 to 2 weeks; then monthly.
- Heparin sodium can be mixed in NS, D_5W, or lactated Ringer's (LR) solution.
- Adjust infusion rates of heparin according to standing orders.
- Use an infusion pump on all heparin infusions.
- Assess your patient's platelet count daily. If it is less than $100,000/mm^3$, notify the prescribing professional immediately.
- After discontinuing heparin and the IV, apply constant pressure to the IV site for at least 5 minutes to stop the bleeding.
- Use of special medication (i.e., topical thromboplastin in a vial) to stop bleeding may be necessary in extreme cases.

Heparin is not compatible with many other drugs, either mixed or Y connected. Check with your pharmacist for compatibility and incompatibility information.

Monitor your patients for complications, such as bleeding from body orifices, especially from the nose and puncture sites (e.g., bone marrow aspiration sites, lumbar puncture sites, IV sites, and laboratory draw sites), and menses flow; hematemesis; hematuria; and black, tarry stools.

Do You UNDERSTAND?

DIRECTIONS: **Answer the following questions.**

1. Mr. Wang is to receive 80 Units/kg of heparin, based on his weight. He weighs 70 kg. What bolus of heparin do you give?
2. Mr. Wang needs to be placed on a heparin drip at 18 Units/kg/hr. His weight is still 70 kg. At how many units per hour should you set the heparin drip?

DIRECTIONS: **Identify the following statements as *True* or *False*.**

3. _____ Heparin dissolves clots.
4. _____ Heparin's dose is calculated according to prothrombin time (PT) laboratory results.
5. _____ Use of NTG with heparin sodium increases heparin's effectiveness.
6. _____ Heparin given by IV infusion requires the use of an IV pump.

Answers: **1. 5600 Units heparin; 2. 1260 Units/hr; 3. False; 4. False; 5. False; 6. True.**

DIRECTIONS: **Fill in the blanks.**

7. A common initial bolus dose of heparin sodium for the treatment of DVT is _____ Units.

8. Therapeutic range of APTT for thromboembolic disease is _____ _____ to _____ times the control value.

9. What hematologic laboratory blood-value count indicates bleeding potential?

What IS Intravenous Nitroglycerin?

IV NTG (e.g., Nitro-Bid, Nitrostat, Tridil) is a parenteral vasodilator that produces peripheral vasodilation, dilates the coronary arteries, and improves blood flow to ischemic areas within the heart. This results in a decrease in myocardial oxygen demand and reduces left ventricular preload and afterload. NTG is used to treat heart failure associated with acute MI. It is also used to treat hypertensive emergencies, angina, and pulmonary edema.

TAKE HOME POINTS

The side effects of NTG include severe headache (mainly occurs during early therapy), flushing of face and neck, dizziness, and postural hypotension.

What You NEED TO KNOW

- NTG IV's onset is 1 to 2 minutes, and its duration is 3 to 5 minutes.
- The initial dose of NTG IV is 2 to 5 mcg/min.
- The use of IV NTG is contraindicated in persons with severe anemia, closed-angled glaucoma, and increased intracranial pressure (ICP) (especially those persons with hypertensive encephalopathy).
- When administering IV NTG to patients, you must closely monitor BP.
- Blood samples from persons on long-term NTG therapy may be chocolate brown in color (because of oxidation of hemoglobin to methemoglobin by the medication).

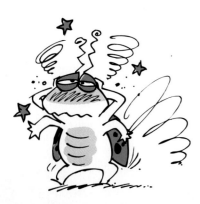

What You DO

- Dilute NTG in D_5W or NS.
- Use an infusion pump with all IV NTG infusions.
- Initially, titrate NTG up by 5 mcg/min every 3 to 5 minutes until the patient's BP responds or you reach a dose of 20 mcg/min. (Further titration is based on patient's response.)
- Three steps can be used to calculate IV NTG flow rate from prescribed doses:
    Step 1: Determine dose per hour.
    Step 2: Convert to like units.
    Step 3: Calculate milliliters per hour (drops/minute).

EXAMPLE: **A patient with heart failure is prescribed IV NTG at 5 mcg/min, and you have 8 mg NTG in 250 ml D_5W in stock. What is the flow rate?**
    Step 1: 5 mcg/min × 60 min = 300 mcg/hr
    Step 2: 300 mcg = 0.3 mg
    Step 3: 8 mg : 250 mL = 0.3 mg : x mL, where x = 9.4 or 9 mL/hr.

- Document onset, type, radiation, location, intensity, and duration of all anginal pain.
- Assess BP and apical pulse before giving NTG.
- Monitor the ECG of all patients receiving IV NTG.
- Assist the patient with ambulation (because of potential dizziness and orthostatic hypotension).
- Wean the patient off IV NTG by decreasing the dose 5 to 10 mcg/min every 10 minutes, while watching for signs of angina or ST segment changes in the ECG.
- A patient's tolerance to IV NTG needs to be built slowly.

TAKE HOME POINTS

- The physical size of a person is no indication of a patient's sensitivity to the drug.
- Drinking alcohol when on NTG will cause the patient to have severe hypotension, vertigo, and pallor.
- Once treatment is complete, patients need to be weaned off of NTG IV.

Do You UNDERSTAND?

DIRECTIONS: **Answer the following questions.**

1. Mr. Showley's prescription reads, "Begin IV Nitrostat titration until it reaches 10 mcg/min. Solution is 8 mg in 250 mL D$_5$W." What is the flow rate in milliliters per hour?

2. Next to each body system, write the name of one condition that can be treated with IV NTG.

   a. Heart: _____

   b. Vascular system: _____

   c. Lungs: _____

3. How does drinking alcohol when using NTG affect a patient's BP?

4. Which electronic-monitoring device is essential to have connected to the patient receiving IV NTG?

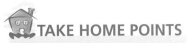

TAKE HOME POINTS

The international normalized ratio (INR) laboratory value decreases in persons on a vitamin K-enriched diet who are receiving anticoagulant therapy.

What IS Vitamin K?

Vitamin K (e.g., AquaMEPHYTON, Konakion, Mephyton) is a fat-soluble vitamin essential in the production of clotting factors. It is used as a nutritional supplement and as an antidote for drug-induced hemorrhage. It is available in tablet or injection form.

What You NEED TO KNOW

Vitamin K is used to:

- Treat biliary disease
- Correct over-coagulation from oral medications (except heparin)
- Decrease bleeding complications in patients who have left ventricular assist devices (LVAD)
- Decrease osteoporosis
- Treat obstructive jaundice

Answers: **1. 19 mL/hr; 2. a. failure or acute MI; b. hypertensive crisis; c. pulmonary edema; 3. it lowers blood pressure; 4. Electrocardiogram (ECG/EKG).**

- A dose of 1 to 2.5 mg of oral vitamin K reduces the international normalized ratio (INR) serum laboratory test value to a therapeutic range within 24 hours in persons receiving the anticoagulant drug warfarin (Coumadin). However, allergic reactions—such as hypotension, rash, sweating, chest pain, bradycardia, and cardiac arrest—can occur in patients receiving vitamin K.
- Antibiotic therapy, especially with broad-spectrum antibiotics, interferes with vitamin K synthesis in the body (leading to the potential for increased bleeding).

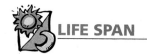

LIFE SPAN

Vitamin K decreases the risk of hip fractures, particularly in older women.
   Vitamin K may be used to treat hemorrhagic states of neonatal patients.

 Monitor patients receiving vitamin K for allergic and hypersensitivity reactions.

What You DO

- Vitamin K can be mixed with preservative-free NaCl or 5% dextrose.
- You should administer vitamin K by IV slowly, at a rate of 1 mg/min.
- Oral doses of vitamin K are 2.5 to 10 mg.
- Monitor laboratory values of PT or INR of persons on anticoagulant medications who may also need vitamin K.
- Assess patients for bruising, petechiae, bleeding gums, hematuria, increased menstrual flow, and bleeding from old puncture sites, and for use of broad-spectrum antibiotics twice a day.
- Use electric razors for shaving and soft toothbrushes for oral care.

TAKE HOME POINTS

- Foods rich in vitamin K include green, leafy vegetables; meat; cow milk; vegetable oil; egg yolks; and tomatoes.
- Instruct your patients to avoid the use of over-the-counter medications unless instructed to take them by their prescribing professional.

Do You UNDERSTAND?

DIRECTIONS: **Select the correct answer.**

1. Vitamin K is given to _____ patient bleeding.
   a. Increase
   b. Decrease

TAKE HOME POINTS

Antibiotic therapy, especially with broad-spectrum antibiotics, interferes with vitamin K synthesis in the body, leading to increased bleeding potential.

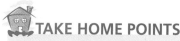**TAKE HOME POINTS**

Vitamin K does not correct over-coagulation resulting from heparin sodium.

Answer: **1. b.**

DIRECTIONS: **Complete the following instructions.**

2. An allergic reaction to vitamin K includes what signs and symptoms?

Cardiac: _____

Blood pressure: _____

Skin: _____

Pain: _____

3. Circle the foods that contain large amounts of vitamin K.

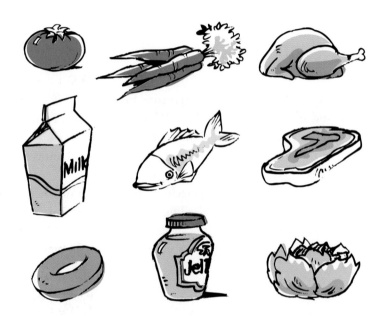

4. What two laboratory values should you assess because they indicate the bleeding time for persons who have the potential to receive vitamin K? _____ and _____

_____

5. Check the category of medications that can interfere with vitamin K synthesis and therefore cause bleeding in patients.

_____ Antibiotics   _____ Cardiac vasodilators

_____ Antihypertensives   _____ Cathartics

_____ Bronchodilators   _____ Diuretics

References

Franco V, Polanczyk CA, Clausell N: Role of dietary vitamin K intake in chronic oral anticoagulation: prospective evidence from observational and randomized protocols, *Am J Med* 116(10):651-6, 2004.

McIntyre KM: Vasopressin in asystolic cardiac arrest, *N Engl J Med* 350(2):179-81, 2004.

Neafsey P: Of blood, bones and broccoli: warfarin-vitamin K interactions, *Home Healthcare Nurs* 1(2):178-84, 2004.

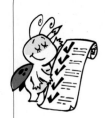

Notes

NCLEX® Review

Circle the correct answer.

1. Dopamine is prescribed at 5 mcg/kg/min. Solution is 250 ml D$_5$W with 400 mg dopamine. Patient weight is 80 kg. What is the flow rate in milliliters per hour?
   1 24 mL/hr
   2 15 mL/hr
   3 24,000 mL/hr
   4 80 mL/hr

2. Nipride is prescribed at 50 mg in 500 mL D$_5$W at 0.8 mcg/kg/min. Patient weight is 65 kg. What is the flow rate in milliliters per hour?
   1 52 mL/hr
   2 1181 mL/hr
   3 62.5 mL/hr
   4 31 mL/hr

3. You are asked to titrate dopamine at 2 to 5 mcg/kg/min to maintain systolic BP greater than 120 mm Hg. Solution is 200 mg dopamine in 500 mL D$_5$W. The patient weighs 62 kg. What are the lower- and upper-flow rates of dopamine in milliliters per hour?
   1 Lower = 121 mL/hr; upper = 184 mL/hr
   2 Lower = 19 mL/hr; upper = 47 mL/hr
   3 Lower = 12 mL/hr; upper = 62 mL/hr
   4 Lower = 11 mL/hr; upper = 88 mL/hr

4. Vasopressin is used during acute hemorrhage from esophageal varices because of what action by this drug?
   1 Contracts smooth muscle
   2 Causes vasoconstriction
   3 Decreases urine flow
   4 Increases renal tubular diuresis

5. Vasopressin is prescribed at 1 Units/mL. You have a 500 mL bag of normal saline in stock. How many units of vasopressin do you add to this NS bag to obtain the prescribed dose?
   1 1
   2 100
   3 500
   4 1000

6. The antidote for heparin sodium is:
   1 Dopamine hydrochloride (Intropin, Dopastat)
   2 Vitamin K (aquaMEPHYTON, Konakion, Mephyton)
   3 Naloxone hydrochloride (Narcan)
   4 Protamine sulfate (Protamine)

7. Mr. Zolinski is to be placed on a heparin drip at 18 Units/kg/hr. He weighs 82 kg. At how many units per hour should you run the heparin drip?
   1 1476
   2 3247
   3 82
   4 4.55

8. Mr. Wadell is admitted to the emergency department in hypertensive crisis. The physician prescribes IV NTG at 8 mcg/min. Solution is 8 mg NTG in 250 mL NS. What is the flow rate?
   1 480 mL/hr
   2 12 mL/hr
   3 15 mL/hr
   4 31 mL/hr

9. What classification of medications does vitamin K counteract?
   1 Anticoagulants
   2 Antidysrhythmics
   3 Opiate narcotics
   4 Antidiarrheals

10. IV vitamin K is normally administered at what rate?
    1 1 mg/min
    2 1 mg/hr
    3 5 mcg/kg/hr
    4 5 mcg/min

11. Short answer: Give one example of a flow rate for intravenous medications. Do NOT give a dose rate.
    _____

12. Fill in the blank: When nitroprusside sodium (Nipride) is used, the patient's cardiac output _____ because there is a decrease in preload and afterload.

13. True or False? Heparin sodium in doses greater than 50,000 Units per day dissolves blood clots in adults.

14. True or False? Headache is a side effect of intravenous nitroglycerin administration.

15. Fill in the blank: A patient on nitroglycerin who also drinks alcohol will experience a _____ in blood pressure.

NCLEX® Review Answers

1. **2** $80 \times 5 = 400$ mcg/min; 400×60 min = 24000 mcg/hr = 24 mg/hr; 400 : 250 = 24 : x, where x = 15 mL/hr.

2. **4** $65 \times 0.8 = 52$; $52 \times 60 - 3120$; 3.12 mg/hr; 50 : 500 = 3.12 : x, where x = 31.2 mL/hr is a lethal dose.

3. **2** Lower = 19 mL/hr; upper = 47 mL/hr

4. **2** Vasoconstriction places pressure on the bleeding areas. Smooth muscle is not that involved in hemorrhage. Urine is not related to the esophagus. Diuresis does not help bleeding from the esophagus.

5. **3** Equal parts means the same amount of drug as fluid. 500 Units.

6. **4** Protamine counteracts the actions of heparin sodium. Dopamine hydrochloride is a sympathomimetic. Vitamin K does not stop bleeding caused by heparin, and naloxone hydrochloride is an antidote for narcotics.

7. **1** $82 \times 18 = 1476$. If you answered 82, you forgot the drip factor. If you answered 4.55, you divided when you should have multiplied.

8. **3** $8 \times 60 = 480 = 0.48$ mg; 8 : 250 = 0.48 : x; $^{120}/_8 = 15$.

9. **1** Anticoagulants counteract bleeding as does vitamin K. Antidysrhythmics counteract heart problems. Opiate narcotics are strong drugs to control pain. Antidiarrheals stop the passage of watery stool.

10. **1** 1 mg/min is the standard flow rate for vitamin K. 1 mg/hr would be too slow to be effective. Micrograms or kilograms are not associated with the administration of vitamin K.

11. mL/hour or gtt/min (drops/minute).

12. Increases.

13. False. Heparin sodium does not dissolve blood clots.

14. True.

15. decrease.

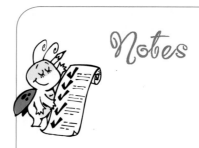

Notes

17

Technology Associated with Drug Administration

What You WILL LEARN

After reading this chapter, you will know how to do the following:
- ✔ Describe the different uses of pumps in patient care.
- ✔ Read and interpret patient prescriptions for medications given via a pump.
- ✔ Calculate rates for medications given by pumps based on prescriptions and patient's clinical condition.

There are many devices, both mechanical and electronic, that use a pumping mechanism to deliver medications and fluids to patients. These devices can be used for intravenous (IV), patient-controlled analgesia (PCA), insulin administration, and for feeding.

What IS an Intravenous Pump?

An *IV pump* is an electronic device for IV medication and fluid delivery. These pumps are either free standing (i.e., they stand alone) or ambulatory (i.e., they are able to be carried). IV pumps work on the principles of gravity or continuous pressure to deliver medications and fluids.

What You NEED TO KNOW

Rate pumps, or gravity pumps, work on the principle of *gravity*. They are designed so that gravity forces the IV fluid into the vein when the IV bag is more than 36 inches above the device's rate controller. A rate controller is an electronic device that regulates IV drip rate. The drop sensor used on the IV tubing counts drops to monitor the desired flow rate in either milliliters per hour or drops per minute, and the drip chamber sounds an alarm when the IV bag is empty.

A pressure pump works on the principle of continuous pressure. They are designed to push IV fluid into the vein at 1 to 9 lb per square inch (psi).

IV pumps are used for:

- The administration of IV fluids and electrolytes, such as D_5W, 20 mEq potassium chloride (KCl), and normal saline (NS) for hydration.
- Hyperalimentation (HPA) (i.e., nutrition that sustains life and maintains growth and development), total parenteral nutrition (TPN) (i.e., nutrition that supplies total caloric needs), and lipids (i.e., fats).
- The administration of baclofen (Lioresal) into the spine to control muscle contractions that cause spasticity (i.e., stiff and awkward movements).
- The administration of opioids, morphine, and hydromorphone (Dilaudid) into the spine to control low-back pain. (This is usually done by implanting a pump beneath the skin.)

There are several things that you should know about IV pumps:

- Each manufacturer of IV pumps has its own special instructions and tubing requirements.
- Most tubing is not interchangeable from manufacturer to manufacturer.
- All pumps need electrical hookups, either for the drip chamber to count drops or for the rate controller to maintain the prescribed rate.
- All pumps have a battery backup that lasts about 3 to 5 hours; it takes about 24 hours to recharge the battery.
- Possible flow rates range from 0.1 to 999.9 mL/hr.
- Pumps have "air-in-line" alarms that sound when more than 100 mcL of air is in the IV line. (A digital readout on the pump alerts the health care provider that air is about to enter the patient's venous system and may cause an air embolism.)
- It takes about 1 to 3 mL of air in the IV tubing (air in more than one third of the entire tubing) to create an air embolism.

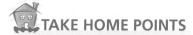

TAKE HOME POINTS

- A rate pump counts drops.
- Gravity is not a factor in using a pressure pump.
- An automatic rate of 20 mL/hr—a keep the vein open (KVO) rate—exists after an alarm is activated.
- A volume pump will continue to force IV fluids, even if the IV is dislodged or out of the vein.

- Normally the body reabsorbs small amounts of air that enters the venous system.
- Pumps have *occlusion* alarms that signal that a blockage has developed somewhere between the IV site and the IV bag when pressure in the IV line exceeds 10 psi. Occlusion can be caused by kinks in the IV tubing, the patient lying on the tubing, or the IV becoming clogged or infiltrated (i.e., out of the vein).
- Some pumps allow you to program them to run a main IV fluid (e.g., 1000 cc NS at 125 cc/hr) and a secondary medication (e.g., antibiotics IV piggyback [IVPB]).
- Most machines have a digital display that allows you to read the total IV intake for your shift (e.g., 7 AM to 3 PM, 3 PM to 11 PM, 11 PM to 7 AM). When working with an IV pump that allows you to monitor IV intake, you must remember to set the display back to "0" after establishing IV intake for your shift. Otherwise the next shift will be counting your shift's intake along with their own.
- Another feature on a few machines is a drug dose calculator that can be used to minimize medication errors. (This is especially helpful in critical-care areas.)

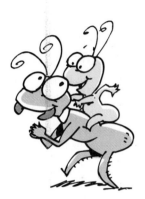

What You DO

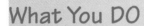

- Assess the patient's need for either a rate or pressure type of IV pump.
- Rate pumps are used when the only concern is that the patient receives specific fluids at specific times (e.g., NS at 100 cc/hour).
- Pressure pumps are used when fluid has to be under pressure to enter the vein, which is usually because the fluid is thick or it is going directly into a pressure-containing organ, such as the heart. Fluid going directly into the heart is administered through a venous access device called a central line.

To use an IV pump to administer medications and fluids:

- Assess the availability of the pump at your institution. (If supply is short, does your patient need one more than other patients in the facility?)
- Assess insurance payment policies regarding the use of an IV pump. (Will insurance cover its use?)
- Evaluate medication, pump prescription, and patient allergies to the medications.

- Plug in the pump and assess it for readiness by examining light indicators.
- Use the recommended tubing and clear it of air by having normal saline move down the tube by gravity.
- Connect the tubing to the machine according to the manufacturer's instructions. (Sometimes clearing the tube requires you to use the action of the machine to push the air out of the line.)
- Attach the tubing to the patient's IV site by screwing the pump tubing onto the IV needle-catheter hub.
- Set the correct rate, volume, and alarm parameters (if indicated) according to the manufacturer's instructions.
- Begin infusion after checking the patient's prescription.
- For the next 5 minutes, assess the IV site for signs of infiltration (e.g., swelling, coolness, and discomfort near the catheter site).
- To ensure that the pump is working correctly, compare the IV rate with the amount of fluid left in the IV bag within 30 to 60 minutes.
- Record administration times on a strip of tape placed on the IV bag so that you can later verify the flow rate.
- Educate your patients, especially outpatients, about the number of hours their IV pump can run on a battery and the number of hours needed to recharge the battery. Also instruct them how to recharge the battery. (This is usually done by plugging it into an electrical outlet for several hours.)

When an alarm sounds, you should check for the following causes (listed in order of occurrence):

- Possible infiltration is occurring at IV site.
- Fluid bag is empty.
- Clamp in IV line is closed.
- Air is in the line.
- Occlusion is occurring.
- Patient position has changed.
- Battery is low.
- Door to IV pump has been left open.
- Flow sensor is dirty or positioned incorrectly.
- Machine is malfunctioning.

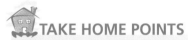**TAKE HOME POINTS**

The use of extension sets (i.e., tubing about 6 inches in length that goes between the IV site and the pump tubing) is not uncommon. Extension sets add to the ease of care.

If infiltration occurs, stop the infusion immediately by clamping the clamp and turning the machine off. Infiltration of certain medications, such as phenytoin (Dilantin), can cause tissue damage.

Periodic biomedical evaluation is required for all pumps. If a pump is not working correctly, remove it from the patient's room and place a sign on it indicating the problem. This will help to prevent another health care provider from using it on another patient before it can be repaired.

Do You UNDERSTAND?

DIRECTIONS: **Fill in the blank.**

1. The principle of gravity is the mainstay of what type of IV pump?

   _____

DIRECTIONS: **Circle the best answer.**

2. Often opioids are used in IV pumps to control:

   High potassium levels   Excess bicarbonate

   Pain   Leg spasms

   Nausea   Diarrhea

DIRECTIONS: **Choose one word from each column to create a phrase to fill in the blanks. (A shape is formed when all the words are connected.)**

3. When the alarm on an IV pump is activated, the rate of the fluid changes to _____ _____ _____.

Gtt	Per	Water
On	Vein	Hours
Normal	Fluid	Saline
Keep	Volume	Open
Potassium	Piggyback	Minute

DIRECTIONS: **Fill in the missing letters in the generic drug name.**

4. What common medication that is used to treat seizures can cause tissue damage if it is injected outside the vein?

   p __ __ n __ t __ i __.

What IS a Syringe Pump?

A *syringe pump* is an IV pump with a motor-driven pressure device and syringe used to administer medications and fluids. This pump is particularly useful for drugs that cannot be mixed with other solutions, such as phenytoin (Dilantin); drugs that need to be given at a controlled rate for a short period of time (i.e., less than 30 minutes); or to minimize fluid given to patients, such as those with renal failure or congestive heart failure (CHF).

What You NEED TO KNOW

Advantages of syringe pumps include:
- Pressure capability is high (up to 78,000 psi), so thick medications can be given and smaller IV tubing, needles, and catheters can be used.
- Maintenance is infrequent. There is not a fluctuating valve such as that found on rate and gravity pumps; as a result, there is no leakage.
- Several syringes can be used in one pump for the administration of multiple medications.
- Pumps are programmable, so more complex protocols can be administered.

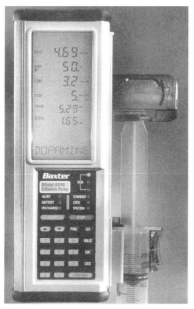

Auto Syringe AS50 Infusion Pump. *Reproduced with permission of Baxter Healthcare.*

Disadvantages of the syringe pump include:
- A limited reserve capacity of 20 to 140 mL.
- The pump is heavy (about 10 lb).

What You DO

- Fill syringe or syringes with drugs and other solutions as prescribed, or obtain prefilled syringes from the pharmacist.
- Verify syringe content and dilution before attaching the syringe to the patient's IV line.

Do You UNDERSTAND?

DIRECTIONS: Select the correct answer.

1. Which of the following patients would benefit from the use of the syringe pump because of the necessity for minimal fluid intake?
   a. A person who has anxiety
   b. A person who has renal failure
   c. A person with chronic obstructive pulmonary disease (COPD)
   d. A person with diabetes mellitus

DIRECTIONS: Circle the correct answer.

2. What is the maximum-reserve capacity of a syringe used in a syringe pump?

10 mL	20 mL
60 mL	100 mL
140 mL	200 mL

DIRECTIONS: Fill in the blank, then answer the question.

3. Mrs. Nagle has had a recent heart attack, and her physician has asked that she not lift or carry anything that weighs over 5 lb. Knowing that the average weight of a syringe pump is _____, should Mrs. Nagle be offered a syringe pump as part of her discharge care?

   _____

What IS a Feeding Pump?

A *feeding pump* is a pressure pump used to control ingestion of gastrointestinal (GI) feedings. This is called enteral nutrition. Feeding pumps are used for patients who have long-term nutritional needs, such as patients who are bedridden or who have Crohn's disease, GI disorders, motility disease, or digestive disorders resulting from cancer surgery. Some pumps provide a flush setting that will automatically flush the tubing so that medications can be fully delivered into the stomach. The flush setting is also used to keep the tube free from clogs.

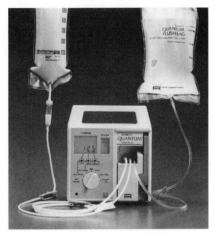

Flexiflo feeding pump. *Reproduced with permission of Ross Products Division, Abbott Laboratories.*

What You NEED TO KNOW

Feeding pumps can be used with many GI tubes, including G-tubes, percutaneous endoscopic gastrostomy (PEG) tubes, and nasogastric (NG) tubes (i.e., tubes that go through the nose and into the stomach), except those tubes with mercury-filled tips (Dobhoff); and jejunostomy tubes (J-tubes), which go directly into the small intestine.

Feeding pump specifics are:
- Battery lasts 8 to 24 hours, if unplugged.
- It takes 5 to 12 hours to recharge the battery.
- Pump weighs 1½ pounds.

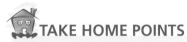

TAKE HOME POINTS

Using a pressure pump or a G-tube that has a mercury-filled tip can cause the mercury to explode into the bloodstream, which will cause mercury poisoning.

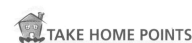

TAKE HOME POINTS

In most cases, residual liquid is usually given back to the patient (rather than being discarded) by pushing it back into the tube immediately after you have pulled it out.

- Range is 1 to 600 mL/hr, with programmable increases of 1 to 10 mL.
- Maximum dose is 3000 mL.
- A display on the pump is available that indicates volume infused.
- Alarm features include: dose completed, no food or empty stomach, occlusion, and low battery.
- Fanny packs are available for some pumps.

What You DO

- Obtain disposable feeding bags and tube sets specific to the pump being used.
- Determine the amount of residual liquid in the stomach, if indicated, by taking a 60 cc (or larger) syringe and pulling back on the syringe once it is connected to the feeding tube to pull out stomach contents. (In most cases, if the residual is more than 50 cc in an adult, the tube feeding is not given. Instead, you should hold the tube feeding for another 2 hours.)
- Often one to two drops of food coloring are added to the feeding to help assess for potential aspiration.
- Place the patient in a sitting position to prevent aspiration and increase digestion, unless contraindicated because of neurologic or hemodynamic problems.
- Change the bags every 12 to 24 hours, depending on the solution being used. Bags need to be changed every 24 hours for infection-control purposes.
- Change bags containing solutions with a high sugar content more frequently because of the increased potential to grow bacteria.
- Periodically assess all tubes for disconnection or leakage.
- Remember that the feeding pump will keep running even if disconnection or leakage occurs.

Do You UNDERSTAND?

DIRECTIONS: Circle and connect the names of tubes that feeding pumps can be used with to treat a patient. The solution is a shape. What shape is it?

1. G   Dobhoff   J
   Hawk   R   DG
   PEG   IG   NG

DIRECTIONS: Select the correct answers.

2. Which of the following statements about a feeding pump is *false*?
   a. The battery lasts 72 hours when it is left unplugged continuously.
   b. The pump weighs 1½ lb.
   c. The display on the pump indicates "volume infused."
   d. The alarm feature includes occlusion.
3. Which sticker is most appropriate to place on every tube feeding bag?
   a. Hazard: radiation
   b. High fructose content
   c. Change bag every 24 hours
   d. Do not shake contents of bag
4. Which of the following patients is most likely to have a feeding pump connected to a feeding tube?
   a. Conscious and walking around
   b. Bedridden for the next 24 hours
   c. Older patient with broken arm; walks to bathroom, requires assistance
   d. Comatose and bedridden for 6 months

Answer: 1. G, J, NG, PEG (forms a rectangle); 2. a; 3. c; 4. d.

What IS a Patient-Controlled Analgesia Pump?

PCA *pump* is a pressure-controlled electronic device that allows the patient to self-administer a prescribed drug for pain control. PCA pumps are used by patients who have severe pain and who need to relieve the temporary pain associated with surgery.

What You NEED TO KNOW

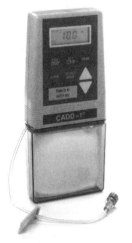

CADD-1 ambulatory pump. *Reproduced with permission of SIMS-Deltec Inc.*

PCA pumps can be set for two types of pain control: (1) a basal rate (i.e., the continuous rate) and (2) a patient-controlled dose. The basal rate is a prescribed rate and dose (sometimes prescribed at zero) that is administered to the patient 24 hours a day. The patient-controlled dose is an extra dose of medication that is available to the patient when it is needed.

Patient-co ntrolled doses allow the patient to push a handheld button that is attached to the machine by a long cord to receive an extra dose of medication. There is a limit to the number of times per hour that the patient can self-medicate, but there is no limit to the number of times the patient can push the button.

Evaluating your patient's pain control is an important responsibility. You should assess the number of times the patient attempts to self-administer pain medication, and keep track of the patient's own pain rating. Doing this will help you to make a clinical judgment as to the effectiveness of pain control prescriptions and procedures.

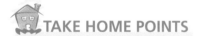

TAKE HOME POINTS

Make sure the patient understands that a PCA pump cannot play "catch-up" to control pain.

What You DO

- Assess the prescription and determine who is legally able to program the pump, usually a registered nurse, a certified registered nurse anesthetist, or a physician.
- Insert a prefilled syringe or bag containing the medication into the PCA device.
- Set the dose, rate, and frequency according to the prescription.

- Record the number of patient self-medication attempts every 4 to 8 hours.
- Obtain the patient's own pain rating using a 1 to 10 scale (10 being severe pain) at least every 4 to 8 hours. If pain relief is not adequate, discuss options with the patient and prescribing professional.
- Monitor vital signs every 1 to 4 hours, especially the patient's respiratory status.

Do You UNDERSTAND?

DIRECTIONS: **Complete the crossword puzzle.**

Down

1. A prescription for morphine sulfate 0.1 mg q1h via PCA. This rate is known as the _____ rate.
2. Something palpable, concrete, or capable of being touched, such as a PCA pump, is a _____ object.
3. Is there a limit to the number of times a patient can push the patient-controlled dose button on a PCA machine?

Across

1. To receive a patient-controlled dose of medication through a PCA pump, the patient must push a handheld _____.
4. Evaluating pain in a patient is known as the fifth vital _____ in nursing.
5. The total dose of medication that the patient can obtain by pushing the button on a PCA pump is called the _____.

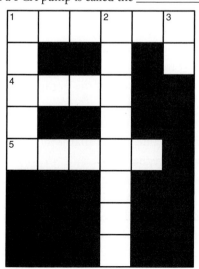

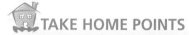
TAKE HOME POINTS

PCA prescription should include:
1. Type of opioid.
2. Dose of opioid.
3. Incremental dose.
4. Delay-time.
5. Maximum dose.
Evaluation of pain is considered the fifth vital sign in nursing.

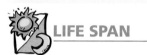
LIFE SPAN

Children rate their pain using a scale based on facial smiles and frowns.
Older patients are less likely to ask for pain medications because they fear they will become addicted or lose their ability to think clearly.
Older patients lack an understanding of the use of the PCA pump and, in general, are afraid of overdosing themselves. Therefore you must take the time to educate them.

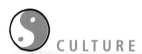
CULTURE

Members of some cultures do not readily admit to pain and must be asked if they are experiencing pain.

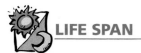

LIFE SPAN

Older patients with memory problems are not candidates for the insulin pump.

TAKE HOME POINTS

- Insulin pumps measure insulin, not blood sugar.
- Glucose-monitoring machines are still required for those who have an insulin pump.

TAKE HOME POINTS

The incidence of type 1 diabetes has increased 3.2% per year over the last decade. The highest incidence occurs in persons ages 0 to 4 years old.

Insulin pump users are at increased risk for diabetic ketoacidosis.

What IS an Insulin Pump?

An *insulin pump* is a small, battery-operated machine that weighs less than 4 oz. Insulin pumps are used to deliver insulin into the body at a constant rate, 24 hours a day, through a needle or cannula (usually placed in the patient's abdomen). An insulin pump can also be programmed to mimic normal insulin secretion, including mealtime requirements.

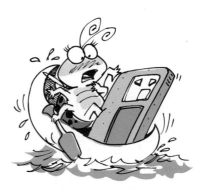

What You NEED TO KNOW

Candidates for an insulin pump include people who:
- Test their blood sugar four or more times a day.
- Have a good knowledge of diabetes.
- Can follow a diet plan.
- Are able to handle the pump technically.
- Are committed to self-care.
- Are able to afford the working cost of the pump (about $1 a day and $5000 to purchase).
- Have a history of hypoglycemic episodes.
- Have a hemoglobin A1C value greater than 7%.
- Are planning to become pregnant.
- Have metabolic instability.
  Advantages of the insulin pump include:
- Tighter control of blood sugars during pregnancy and in general.
- Precision (delivers as little as 0.1 Units of insulin).
- Flexibility (increases quality of life by eliminating insulin injections).

- Have increased control: allows more flexibility during mealtimes, carbohydrate intake, and exercise levels; delays the onset of diabetic retinopathy (eye damage), nephropathy (kidney damage), and neuropathy (nerve damage).

There are several things that you should know about insulin pumps:

- The placement site of the needle or cannula should be changed every 2 to 3 days (either by the health care provider or patient).
- The needle or cannula should always be placed into subcutaneous (SC) tissue (e.g., upper buttocks, abdomen, upper arms, thighs, and upper back).
- The batteries need to be changed every 8 weeks. (There is an alarm feature on the pump that notifies you when the batteries are running low.)
- The ability to adjust insulin delivery is helpful in preventing hypoglycemia during sleep.
- Although most pumps use regular insulin, there are some that use lispro (Humalog, human insulin rDNA) insulin, which has a more rapid onset than regular insulin and a shorter duration of action.

Common Insulin Pump Insulins

Lispro–rapid acting.
Aspart–rapid acting.
Regular–short acting.

- To program the machine to cover insulin requirements before each meal, the patient will still need to take a blood sugar reading using a glucose-monitoring machine.
- Most pumps are watertight, so there is no need to worry if the patient gets the device wet. When taking a shower, the patient uses a specifically designed, plastic shower bag to protect the pump.
- Some insulin pumps have the capability of releasing the ½-inch tubing from the pump so that the patient can get dressed.
- When bathing, the patient should set the pump on the floor or on a suction cup on the shower door.
- For swimming or during intimacy, most people temporarily disconnect the pump. Some pumps (Animas) can be used in a swimming pool.
- For sports, there is a special guard for the pump.
- Pump alarms include: low battery, empty reservoir of insulin, and occlusion.

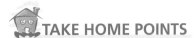

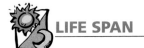

LIFE SPAN

During growth spurts in adolescents, additional insulin is required because the growth hormone promotes insulin resistance.

- On average, pump repairs are needed every 8 years.
- Most insurance companies cover insulin pumps. Precertification is required.
- Insulin pumps are not affected by electromagnetic interference from radios, portable telephones, or microwave ovens.

What You DO

- Be sure that your patient knows the insulin pump's alarm alert sensitivity. Some pumps are designed to sound an alarm if 2 Units of insulin are missed; others sound an alarm when 4 Units are missed.
- Make sure the patient knows the type of batteries that the pump takes (3 or 1.5 volt) and whether the pump displays the time in military time or AM and PM time.
- Patients using an insulin pump should know how often the machine self-checks. If the self-check is unsuccessful, an alarm will sound and the problem will be listed on the pump's screen.
- The patient should also know the length of the pump's warranty, which averages 2 to 4 years.
- Anyone using an insulin pump should be checked for allergies to pork, beef, or the type of insulin prescribed.
  To install an insulin pump:
- Wash the skin site with soap and water or alcohol and allow it to air dry.
- Using sterile technique, insert the infusion-set needle into subcutaneous tissue.
- Apply an antibiotic ointment if the patient is prone to skin infections.
- Cover with bioclusive dressing or sterile 2 × 2 (tape around all four sides of the dressing).
- Program the pump, as prescribed.
- Place the pump in the patient's pocket, bra, or special case worn on a belt.
- Assess the site for signs of infection every 2 to 4 hours, and keep track of alternating sites.
- Teach the patient how to fill the insulin cartridge or reservoir and how to change the infusion set.
- Show the patient how to administer a bolus of insulin for meals and how to change the basal rate when involved in a physical activity.

• Discuss possible pump problems, and explain to the patient how to fix them (see table below).

Insulin Pump Problems and Solutions

Problems	Solutions
Hub leaks	Tighten firmly or replace the hub if it smells of insulin.
Insulin crystallizes and occludes infusion	Remove infusion from site, replace infusion set, and restart in another area. Give prescribed bolus of insulin.
O-ring leaks	Relubricate pump barrel by freeing it from the reservoir and pushing the plunger all the way into the reservoir to pick up some lubricant. Then pull it back to the reservoir to put air into the insulin bottle.
Site bleeds excessively or a hematoma forms	Remove infusion from site. If a hematoma has formed, pinch the lump under the skin and remove as much fluid as possible. Apply warm compresses. Restart infusion in another area. Assess the patient's temperature every 4 hours for 12 hours.
Extensive sweating makes the needle fall out	Apply odorless, antibacterial antiperspirant to the infusion site. Use a liquid adhesive or bioclusive skin dressing.

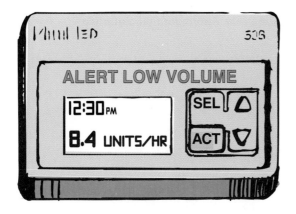

Do You UNDERSTAND?

DIRECTIONS: **Circle the number of hours per day that regular insulin is pumped into the patient's body using an insulin pump.**

1. 4　　6　　10　　12　　18　　24

DIRECTIONS: **One of the advantages of using an insulin pump is that it helps prevent the onset of several diabetic-induced conditions. Write the name of the associated diabetic condition under each picture.**

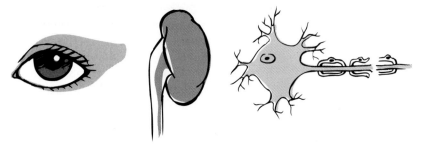

2. _____ _____ _____

DIRECTIONS: **Place an X on all the body parts.**

3. In what subcutaneous areas on the front of the body can a needle or cannula for an insulin pump be inserted?

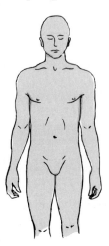

DIRECTIONS: **Fill in the blank.**

4. The ability to adjust insulin delivery is very helpful in preventing low blood sugar, which occurs during sleep. Another name for low blood sugar is _____.

DIRECTIONS: **Circle the correct answer.**

5. Which one of the following energy sources does an insulin pump use?

   Solar   Battery   Nuclear   Electric

DIRECTIONS: **Circle the correct picture.**

6. The use of warm compresses on the SC needle or cannula insertion site is recommended for what possible problem caused by an insulin pump?

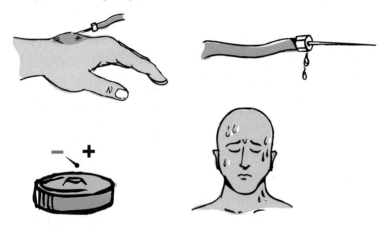

References

Gross TM, Kayne D, King A et al:. A bolus calculator is an effective means of controlling postprandial glycemia in patients on insulin pump therapy, *Diabetes Technol Ther* 5(3):365-9, 2003.

Mottershaw M. Could insulin pump therapy benefit preschool children? *J Diabetes Nurs* 7(6):219-21, 2003.

Reiff PA, Niziolek MM: Troubleshooting tips for PCA, *RN* 64(4):33-7, 2001.

Tucker C: The insulin pump specialty, *Diabetes Educator* 30(2):232, 234, 2004.

Answers: 4. **hypoglycemia; 5. Battery; 6. Hematoma.**

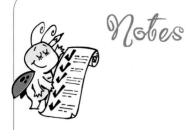

Notes

NCLEX® Review

Circle the correct answer.

1. Your patient, who is moderately hypertensive, is prescribed lipids at 15 mL/hr. Because the prescription calls for a thick fluid, an IV pump that can push fluid into the vein is required. What type of IV pump should be used?
   1 Pressure pump
   2 Rate pump
   3 Gravity pump
   4 Solar pump

2. Your patient has been walking the halls and visiting with relatives in the visitor's area for almost 5 hours. His IV pump begins to sound an alarm. What is the most likely cause of the alarm?
   1 The flow sensor is not positioned correctly.
   2 The machine has malfunctioned.
   3 There is a closed clamp on the IV line.
   4 The battery is low.

3. Your patient, Mrs. Gondales-Remerez, needs to be given a medication at a controlled rate over 90 minutes. Is the syringe pump a good choice?
   1 Yes
   2 No
   3 Only physicians can give medications using a syringe pump.
   4 Syringe pumps are not used to give medications.

4. One of the disadvantages of a syringe pump is that it:
   1 Requires frequent maintenance
   2 Is not programmable
   3 Can only hold one syringe per pump
   4 Has a limited reserve capacity

5. Your patient's G-tube becomes disconnected from the machine's feeding tube. What will the feeding pump do under these circumstances?

   1 It will shut off automatically.
   2 It will keep on pumping.
   3 The alarm will go off because it has detected an occlusion.
   4 It will slow to the KVO rate.

6. You set your patient's feeding pump to infuse the total 100 mL of an enteral tube feeding. The alarm beeps at the infusion amount of 101 mL. The alarm most likely indicates:
   1 Occlusion
   2 No food or empty stomach
   3 Low battery
   4 Dose completed

7. The prescription for a patient's patient-controlled analgesia (PCA) pump reads, "Morphine sulfate 0.1 mg basal rate, plus patient-controlled dose of 0.1 mg q4h." What is the total dose of morphine allowed in a 24-hour period?
   1 24 mg
   2 2.4 mg
   3 2.8 mg
   4 3 mg

8. PCA pumps require you, as a health care provider, to set the pump. The settings should include the medication dose, rate, and which of the following.
   1 Amount
   2 Frequency
   3 Number of attempts
   4 Pain-relief range of scores

9. Mrs. Wattington has had her insulin pump for 8 weeks when an alarm sounds. What is the most likely cause of the alarm?
   1 Occlusion has occurred.
   2 The pump needs to be repaired.
   3 The battery is low.
   4 The clamp is still clamped on the IV tubing.

10. Which of the following statements is proof that a patient does not understand how to use their insulin pump?
    1 "Now I do not need to check my blood sugar anymore."
    2 "I need to change my SC insertion site every 2 to 3 days."
    3 "I still can take a shower."
    4 "My insulin pump uses regular insulin."

11. Your patient is prone to skin infections. For site care, you recommend:
    1 Scrubbing the site with bleach
    2 Applying aloe plant extract
    3 Applying a paste made of equal parts of vinegar and baking soda
    4 Applying antibiotic ointment

12. True or False? Gravity is a factor in using a pressure pump for intravenous administration of medications.

13. True or False? A disadvantage of a syringe pump for intravenous administration of medications is a limited reserve capacity.

14. Short answer: What is added to tube feedings to assist in assessing for potential aspiration? _____

15. Fill in the blank: What is the name used to describe the continuous rate of a patient-controlled analgesia (PCA) pump? The _____ rate.

NCLEX® Review Answers

1. **1** A pressure pump pushes lipids into the vein. A rate pump just counts drops. Gravity does not help thick liquids flow into the vein, and there is no solar pump available.

2. **4** Battery life is usually 3 to 5 hours. If the flow sensor was positioned incorrectly, the machine malfunctioned, or there was a closed clamp on the IV line, an alarm would have sounded early on.

3. **2** Only medications given for less than 30 minutes are choices for syringe pumps. Because the medication is to be administered for over 30 minutes, the syringe pump is not a good choice. Nurses can give medications by syringe pump.

4. **4** Has a limited reserve capacity. The capacity is 20 to 140 mL for a syringe pump. Maintenance is about twice a year for a syringe pump, and such a pump is programmable. Several syringes can be held at one time on a syringe pump.

5. **2** Because there is no obstruction, it is probably being pumped into the patient's bed. The machine does not have the capability to shut off automatically, and there is no occlusion, so an alarm will not sound. Slowing to KVO rate occurs when there is no fluid left in the bag.

6. **4** The alarm indicates dose completed because there is no fluid left in the bag. There is not a "no food" or "empty stomach" alarm on a feeding pump. If an alarm for low battery sounded, this would be a coincidence.

7. **4** $(0.1 \times 24 \text{ hours} = 2.4)$ plus $(0.1 \times {}^{24}/_4 = 0.6)$; $2.4 + 0.6 = 3.0$.

8. **2** How often is very important, and dose means the same as amount. Attempts can occur as often as the patient chooses. Pain relief range of scores is not a setting, but it is a fifth vital sign.

9. **3** Batteries last about 6 to 8 weeks. Occlusions can occur anytime. A repair is highly unlikely. The alarm will sound on the first day of use if there is still a clamp on the IV tubing.

10. **1** Blood sugar still needs to be checked. Changing the SC insertion site every 2 to 3 days is appropriate. Showers are permitted. Insulin pumps use regular insulin.

11. **4** Antibiotic ointment prevents and helps ease skin infections. Scrubbing the site with bleach is very irritating to the skin, and aloe is used to reduce

itching, not infections. A vinegar and baking soda paste has no antiinfection properties.

12.   False.

13.   True. Reserve capacity is 20 to 140 mL.

14.   Food coloring.

15.   basal.

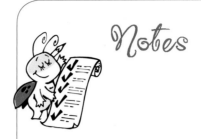

Index

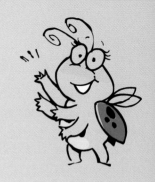